ME
TOO

First published in the United States of America in 1995 by WRS Publishing, A division of WRS Group, Inc., 701 N. New Road, Waco, Texas 76710
Book design by Yvonne Chiu
Jacket design by Joe James

10 9 8 7 6 5 4 3 2 1

Library of Congress Cataloging-in-Publication Data

Payne, James E., 1935-
    Me too: a doctor survives prostate cancer / James E. Payne.
              p.   cm.
    ISBN 1-56796-086-3 (PB)
    1. Payne, James E., --1935- --Health. 2. Prostate--Cancer--Patients--
Biography.   I. Title.
RC280.P7P39   1995
362.1'9699463'0092--dc20
[B]
                                                        95-18870
                                                        CIP

ME
TOO

A Doctor Survives Prostate Cancer

JAMES E. PAYNE, M.D.

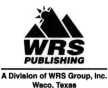

WRS
PUBLISHING

A Division of WRS Group, Inc.
Waco, Texas

To my wife, Linden,
who was always there for me

ACKNOWLEDGMENT

To my former student, longtime friend, and outstanding urologist Dr. Joseph L. Williams, whose empathetic medical management and skillful surgical treatment were paramount in my successful recovery from prostate cancer. In addition, Joe spent considerable time and effort reviewing my manuscript to assure I didn't say something dumb about the various urologic procedures I describe.

PREFACE

Actors Don Ameche and Bill Bixby, rock music star Frank Zappa, and 35,000 other men died of prostate cancer in the United States in 1993. In 1994, Telly Savalas and Thomas P. (Tip) O'Neill succumbed to the effects of this disease. In addition, my personal friends Blackie Moake and Sid Lanier were recently diagnosed with prostate cancer. So were my personal physician's brother, two co-workers, my wife's friend's husband, and a retired, former commander in the Air Force. Prominent personalities Roger Moore and Robert Goulet, Senator Robert Dole of Kansas, and King Sihanouk of Cambodia have undergone treatment for prostate cancer; and, more recently, retired Army General Norman Schwarzkopf, Desert Storm commander. It seems I hear about someone having prostate cancer almost weekly. It is really that prevalent!

Prostate cancer is the most common cancer in men except minor skin cancer. Its death rate has increased slowly but steadily since 1962. By 1990, prostate cancers were claiming the lives of 25 of 100,000 American men each year. Today, it is the second leading cause of cancer death in men. In 1994 in the U.S., 200,000 new cases of prostate cancer were diagnosed, and more than 38,000 men died of the effects of this capricious malignancy.

The diagnostic procedures available for prostate cancer testing have changed in the last few years. Until recently, many prostate cancers were not diagnosed until they were large enough to produce symptoms, usually pain from cancer spread to bones. Some were detected early by digital rectal examination, but many of these were advanced also. In elderly men, many prostate cancers were discovered hidden in tissue removed at operations for benign prostatic hyperplasia (BPH) symptoms. Prostate cancers discovered in this manner are the least likely to behave aggressively. In fact, many of these never cause symptoms, either local or due to metastases. These two diagnostic extremes—very advanced, or in the very elderly—may have skewed our expectations for treatment or our predictions of how prostate cancer behaves.

Today, because of the availability of the prostate specific antigen (PSA) blood test, physicians can diagnose prostate cancer much earlier. If the test is used correctly and efficaciously, the mortality rate should improve for younger men, who develop the more virulent, faster-growing type of prostate cancer. But to date, the potential of the PSA has not been realized. In fact, some medical authorities fear that early detection of prostate cancer will result in unnecessary radical treatment. They worry that the treatment will cause more death and disability than would the cancer itself. Dr. Stephen Goldfinger, editor of the *Harvard Health Letter,* wrote recently, "In the stage where prostate cancer can be detected only in this way [prostate specific antigen testing], it grows so slowly that you will almost always die of something else first—and the surgery can really do a number on you [causing considerable discomfort and possibly impairing sexual function]."

The treatment of newly diagnosed prostate cancer is controversial. Most authorities recommend radical extirpative surgery if the cancer is localized and the patient is young and healthy enough to withstand a major operation. Unfortunately, this treatment is most likely to cause physiological changes that adversely affect a younger man's physical and psychological well-being. Specifically, irreversible sexual impotence is the result in most cases. And disabling urinary incontinence occurs more than infrequently. These, and other less common side effects of "successful" treatment, can be devastating to a man even if the surgery is curative. Primary radiation therapy is also associated with significant complications, including impotence. Radiation is usually better tolerated by older men than is radical surgery, however, and the results of treatment are comparable.

Prostate cancer is a puzzling disease in many respects. There is no known cause, but it is three times more prevalent in men who have a family history of prostate cancer. Advanced age is the single most common risk factor, however. About 80 percent of prostate cancers are diagnosed in men over the age of sixty-five. The disease is uncommon in men under fifty. It is also more common in blacks, and their survival rate is poorer, irrespective of treatment and stage of the disease. Some welders and workers who are involved in electroplating or alkaline battery production and who have been shown to have increased exposure to cadmium have a higher incidence of prostate cancer. Also, occupational exposure to rubber has been implicated in the development of the disease. No one knows why. Diets high in animal fats, polysaturated oils, and animal sources of dietary protein have been linked to increased risk of prostate cancer, but the relationship of diet and the disease is unclear.

My prostate cancer was a complete surprise. I was a full seven years short of age sixty-five at the time of my diagnosis. No one in my Caucasian family had had prostate cancer, including my father who died at eighty-seven. I had no symptoms, and my digital rectal examination was completely normal.

A man over age fifty must be concerned about prostate cancer. In the U.S., one in eleven of us will get it. If you must personally fight this cancer, or if someone you love develops prostate cancer, I hope the following account will be of value to you in your struggle.

CHAPTER 1

Never trouble trouble till trouble troubles you.
                                                    –Anonymous

I'm gonna live 'til I die!
I'm gonna keep flyin' high!
I'm gonna fill my cup until my number's up,
I'm gonna live, live, live until I die!

                              —Kent, Curtis, and Hoffman
                              "I'm Gonna Live Until I Die"

To begin at the beginning: My world began to unravel Friday, February 7, 1992, eight days before my fifty-seventh birthday. One week earlier, I had undergone a routine yearly physical examination by my internist, Dr. Judy Williamson, a staff internist at Bergstrom Air Force Base, Texas. Judy had been treating my medical problems for over a year as if I were her father. She may have actually considered me a father figure, since the age difference was sufficient. Also, she remembered me as her commander, Air Force Colonel Payne, during her residency training years.

A year after I retired from the Air Force to take my present position with the Texas Rehabilitation Commission, I developed mild but persistent diastolic hypertension. The Bergstrom Hospital commander, another former student of mine during his medical training, referred me to Dr. Bill McLeod, chief of internal medicine, to treat my high blood pressure. During my clinic appointments, Dr. Williamson and I would frequently exchange pleasantries. She would occasionally treat me if Dr. McLeod was busy or unavailable. When Dr. McLeod left the Air Force, Dr. Williamson became my primary physician. Judy seemed truly grateful to be my doctor, and she never missed an opportunity to do an indicated examination or recommended test.

Dr. Williamson called me at my office in late January to remind me (as if I needed reminding) that my birthday was approaching. She and I needed to arrange my annual physical examination and associated routine tests. We did that. After finding all systems normal on examination, she decided that I should have my first prostate specific antigen test (PSA), a relatively new blood test for prostate cancer screening.

Late in the afternoon of Friday, February 7, I had arrived home after a busy work-week and was sipping my customary TGIF martini when Judy called.

"Dr. Payne, I got the results of your blood tests back and everything was okay except that your PSA was slightly elevated. It probably doesn't mean a thing, but I think we ought to get a urology consultation to evaluate your prostate. I hope this news doesn't spoil your weekend."

"Not at all, Judy. I appreciate your interest and concern. By all means, let's proceed with the urology consult."

Translation: Not only have you spoiled my weekend, but every day and night for the foreseeable future until some knowledgeable specialist can truthfully say, Well, Dr. Payne, we've run every test, X-ray, scan, and gadgetry known to God and man, and we find that your only possible problem is an overactive libido. Further, although each test was extremely uncomfortable, expensive, and completely dehumanizing, and the normal findings were reported agonizingly slowly, we declare you healthy and free of any forms of cancer.

But that wasn't to be, and I think I knew that from the very beginning.

CHAPTER 2

God never built a Christian strong enough to carry today's duties and tomorrow's anxieties piled on the top of them.

—Theodore Ledyard Cuyler

Sunday, February 9, was a beautiful springlike day in Austin, Texas. My wife, Linden, and I had tickets to a play at a local theater that happened to be in a very attractive park area of the city. As we drove to the theater I spoke disparagingly about a gaudy fast-food cafe being built near the park. I expounded my opinion about its bad effect on the ambience of the area. Linden blandly expressed her disagreement with my point of view, and, surprisingly, it made me absolutely furious with her. I exploded with a terrible tirade. She was shocked at my outburst, and understandably so, since we had developed an almost perfect relationship over our thirty-plus years of happy marriage based on mutual respect. We seldom had unpleasant words.

My bad humor continued at a slow burn through most of the humorless comedy we were watching. I didn't regain my complete composure until I walked out in the middle of the play and left the theater. I watched a pickup softball game in an adjacent ball field until the play was over. Only then, in the peace and warmth of the lovely day, did my rage mellow into a blue funk. Tomorrow, Monday, I must call a urologist to schedule an appointment for an early examination.

Earlier that week Dr. Williamson asked me if I had a urologist of choice. Upon learning I had none, she suggested Dr. Joe Williams, a local civilian urologist with whom she had developed a good professional relationship. Dr. Williams spent a morning a week at the Bergstrom Hospital as a urology consultant to the Air Force physicians. I remembered Joe from his training days at Wilford Hall Medical Center in the late 1970s. Then, I was clinical director of the Wilford Hall general surgery residency program. He had rotated through general surgery for two years as a pre-urology resident under my supervision. How could I turn down the services of a surgeon I had helped train? He must be great!

When I telephoned Dr. Williams Monday, he remembered me and was very kind and encouraging. He assured me that with my mild but progressive benign prostatic hyperplasia (BPH) symptomatology, a PSA of 5.8 nanograms per milliliter was not a biggie. We scheduled an examination and probable transrectal prostate ultrasound for Wednesday, February 12.

On the day of my appointment, Dr. Williams explained to me that BPH commonly causes minor elevations of PSA. Transrectal ultrasound can accurately estimate the volume of one's prostate in grams. With the known prostate volume, we can calculate a PSA/prostate gland ratio. If there is less than .15 or so nanograms of PSA per gram of prostate, malignancy is unlikely to be the reason for the elevated PSA. This is assuming a normal digital prostate examination, of course, and no ultrasound irregularities. Dr. Williams exuded confidence and optimism that this would be the case with me.

Matt, Dr. Williams' technical assistant, was a large, early-middle-aged man who was pleasant, self-assured, and very professional. A former Air Force medic, he left the service to work for Dr. Williams in civilian practice. As Matt set up instruments and prepared me for the study, he tried to reassure me about the safety and ease of ultrasound-guided transrectal biopsy of the prostate. I told him I had just as soon they not find anything worth a biopsy. Matt quickly agreed, but I got the distinct impression that it would be unusual for Dr. Williams to walk away from this procedure without a specimen for a pathologist to examine microscopically.

Dr. Williams first did a digital rectal examination (ugh!) and assured me that my prostate felt perfectly smooth, but smaller than he expected. He then went on with the ultrasound examination. This involved placement of a solid metal tubular probe into my rectum that felt not unlike the difficult passage of a constipated stool—not really painful, but distinctly uncomfortable. Joe kept up a running dialogue of what he was doing and why. He described what he termed a mildly suspicious area of the right lobe ("hypoechoic" by ultrasound) that apparently would require a biopsy, to my chagrin. Using a spring-loaded biopsy needle and guided by an ultrasound image, Dr. Williams made three quick biopsies. This proved to be another new experience I would have preferred to forego, but an interesting sensation in a perverse sort of way. Coincidental with Dr. Williams' explanation that I would feel pressure and "a little stick," I did actually feel pressure, then a gradual sharp, localized pain. It quickly dissolved into the dull ache characteristic of visceral pain. The sensation was like the discomfort of a prostate digital examination, but much more subtle and, surprisingly, quite short-lived.

"I see nothing else abnormal anywhere on ultrasound, Dr. Payne, but I'm going to take one random biopsy from the left lobe for staging. I do this routinely on everyone," Joe stated.

Thanks a lot! I murmured quietly to myself.

Afterward, in his office, Dr. Williams showed me the photographs of the ultrasound examination and the "suspicious" area of the right side. "It's not at all impressive, but it's the only abnormal area I saw. I'd estimate maybe a 20 percent chance it will turn out to be anything significant. But your prostate was surprisingly small—only 17 grams. I expected it to be considerably larger." He continued, very upbeat, "I know you're concerned, and I would be, too. I'm sorry we couldn't put this to rest today, but I still think everything is going to turn out negative; and believe me, as soon as I get the good word from the pathologist, I'll call you immediately."

A few minutes later Joe did another final rectal digital examination to assure that no subcapsular bleeding from the biopsies had developed to form a hematoma (collection of blood). He scheduled a follow-up appointment for the following Tuesday, February 18. "It generally takes five to six work days for the pathologist to get his report back to my office," he told me.

Sure, I thought to myself, as I drove home, but if you're concerned, you can get a report by telephone in three days—four days max.

While driving home I kept waiting for side effects from my ordeal to begin—the development of excruciating pelvic pain, at least. This might be indicative of a prostatic hemorrhage that would require emergency surgery. Perhaps I would develop chills and fever followed by septic shock, hematuria, seizures, and loss of consciousness. That would probably cause an auto accident, undoubtedly involving a bus loaded with orphan children on their way to an outing. Oh, brother! I thought to myself. With my textbook knowledge of surgical disease and treatment complications, I was going to make one helluva great patient.

CHAPTER 3

He is the best physician who is the most ingenious inspirer of hope.

—Samuel Taylor Coleridge

Saturday, February 15, I "celebrated" my fifty-seventh birthday. Except for my preoccupation with my new physical infirmity possibilities, it would have been a pleasant and relaxing day. Linden cooked me a very enjoyable dinner, and she and I had an intimate, private birthday party. I received birthday cards and telephone calls from my children and grandchildren wishing me a happy birthday and expressing their love. Unfortunately, my mind was so focused on my fear of having cancer, I was barely touched by their attention.

My biopsy report would be available Monday, February 17. If it was negative I was certain I would get a congratulatory call from Dr. Williams sometime that day. He didn't call, so I knew instinctively the news was bad.

When I arrived for my appointment Tuesday, February 18, the office receptionist and Matt were pleasant, but distant and aloof. (They knew!) While sitting in the waiting room, I caught a glimpse of Dr. Williams behind the reception desk area. Our eyes met and he quickly looked away. Presently, I was ushered directly into the doctor's office. Dr. Williams entered promptly, loud and in good humor, as usual. He greeted me cordially, sat down behind his large desk, and got right to the point: The biopsies of the hypoechoic area of the right lobe were negative for cancer, but the random staging biopsy of the left lobe, surprisingly, showed cancer—adenocarcinoma. Pathologically, it was a Gleason grade 6 (moderate cell differentiation).

We talked at length about prostate cancer and its

capricious nature. Usually an indolent cancer in the elderly (over age seventy or so), it can occasionally be very aggressive and rapidly fatal, especially in younger men (my age and below).

If Joe Williams hadn't chosen a career in medicine, he would have been great in the diplomatic corps. Although I was devastated by his confirmation that I had been inducted into the dreaded fraternity of "The Big C," Joe's optimistic demeanor almost made me feel fortunate to have been chosen. "How lucky to have discovered the tumor at this early stage, Dr. Payne! By all indications, it's an extremely early cancer. It's not palpable, it's localized, and it's asymptomatic! Fortuitously, we've diagnosed a potentially lethal tumor before it has had a chance to spread and become incurable!" Dr. Williams beamed. "Why, only last night I was reading an article by one of the world's leading authorities on prostate cancer," he continued, "and this article recommended that with findings such as yours, they would do nothing! No ultrasound, no biopsy, nothing! Only repeat your PSA in a year."

We discussed treatment: surgery versus radiation. For prostate cancer localized to the gland, statistical results by either modality are about the same for the first ten years. Then, the incidence of recurrence and metastases in the radiation treatment group begins to rise much faster than in the radical surgery treatment group.

"You're a young man, Dr. Payne. Because you have many more than ten years of quality life to look forward to, I think you should have surgery—a radical retropubic prostatectomy. If you were seventy-five years old, I'd probably not consider surgery and opt for radiation."

My recollection of radical prostatectomies from the days when I was a professor of surgery (and Dr. Williams was a surgery resident) was not a favorable one. I recalled five- or six-hour-long, bloody, uncontrolled operations associated with multiple complications and high mortality. Dr. Williams explained that the art had much advanced since then. With improved anatomic definition of the pelvic vasculature and updated surgical techniques, there had been substantial improvement in the operative complication rate. Further, advancement in anesthesia had made the procedure safer from possible pulmonary complications and much less painful postoperatively. Even the nerves that control sexual potency had been better defined. And it was likely that, with my localized disease, a nerve-sparing procedure could be accomplished to potentially preserve potency without compromising the chances for a complete cure. Dr. Williams had gained extensive experience in the last few years using this advanced procedure for his prostate cancer patients. A young associate who trained under the urologist who pioneered these newest techniques routinely assisted him at operation.

Dr. Williams went on to explain that the first step of the operation would be to sample the retroperitoneal pelvic lymph glands that drain the prostate. Several would be excised for frozen section examination by the pathologist at surgery. If metastatic tumor was found, Dr. Williams would abort the operation. That would show that the tumor had extended beyond the scope of surgery. Later, external beam radiation therapy could be used to treat the tumor. But if the frozen section examination was negative, he would go on with the radical prostatectomy. This operation included removal of the prostate, seminal vesicles, and the adjacent pelvic lymph glands—a curative procedure.

In years past I had often speculated on what to do if I needed serious medical treatment, generally meaning major surgery (and usually thinking coronary artery bypass). I had always assumed I would use my knowledge and professional status to seek out the top authority in the field and push whatever buttons necessary to secure his (her?) services. Surprisingly, not only had Dr. Williams sold me on surgery versus radiation (truthfully, I had always feared the thought of surgery!), but he had convinced me I would do no better under the scalpel of any other surgeon.

Doctors universally hate and fear treating other doctors, despite what is depicted in the movies or on TV. Not only are doctors generally lousy patients— hostile to the nursing personnel, disruptive, and dictatorial—but they're a sure bet to invoke Murphy's Law during treatment: If anything can possibly go wrong, it will. Or to paraphrase: If any complication can possibly happen during the treatment of a doctor, it inevitably will, and will be the worst one you have ever seen.

My only question to Dr. Williams was whether he would feel uncomfortable performing my surgery and being the physician responsible for my treatment. His answer was touching, and convincing. "I would feel perfectly comfortable performing your operation, Dr. Payne. I appreciate what you've done for me in the past, and I'd like to think that I had a part in making it possible for us to be friends and associates for many more years to come."

But first I had to pass several qualifying tests to be considered a candidate for curative surgery. And now I had a new set of unknown devils to occupy my mind.

CHAPTER 4

The world is so full of care and sorrow that it is a gracious debt we owe to one another to discover the bright crystals of delight hidden in somber circumstances and irksome tasks.

—Helen Keller

Several weeks earlier, Linden and I had enrolled in a night class at the University of Texas that we attended Tuesdays and Thursdays. The class, American Sign Language, was great fun and quite educational, and interacting with hearing-impaired clients was a big part of my job. We especially enjoyed walking on campus to class pretending we were young college kids again.

We went to class as usual that Tuesday evening after I arrived home from Dr. Williams's office. Because of the hustle and bustle to get to class on time, Linden and I didn't have time to talk, so I made no reference to my visit with Dr. Williams. After class, I remembered nothing about the lesson. My mind was too full of self-concern about my diagnosis—and how and when to tell Linden that I had prostate cancer.

After Linden and I arrived back home from class I quickly poured myself three fingers of Jack Daniels. We sat ourselves on the sofa in the living room and I told my wife about my test results as matter-of-factly as I could. Linden is a strong lady, and she took the news well—really too well, I thought. I wondered if she understood that in a few weeks I would be dead or dying of a cancer that was spreading through my body like hot syrup over pancakes. Although I knew that prostate carcinoma didn't behave that way, my mind wasn't functioning on its highest level by any means. It wouldn't for some time.

Upon the revelation of my diagnosis, Linden reacted

more with belligerence than any other emotion I expected, such as sadness, remorse, pity, or fear. This surprised me a bit, but I probably wouldn't have been satisfied with any emotion short of a grand mal seizure. I had enough self-pity for her and several other people. Later, I thought how typical it was of Linden to get angry and ready to fight this threat to her lover—a more positive emotion than I was experiencing, and healthier, too. Even after all these years she continued to impress me with her emotional strength.

CHAPTER 5

How much have cost us the evils that never happened!

–Thomas Jefferson

When a patient is diagnosed with any kind of cancer, it's necessary next to determine whether there is evidence of metastasis, a spreading of the tumor beyond the primary site. This is especially true if extirpative surgery (complete excision) is a consideration. Various tests—radioisotope scans, organ function studies, imaging, X-rays—are helpful in deducing evidence of metastasis. Such tests are largely low risk or risk-free to the patient (but not exactly "free" in a monetary sense!), and they provide extremely important information. For example, a radical colon resection with creation of a colostomy stoma might cure a localized cancer of the rectum. But this dangerous operation, with all its inherent risks and lifestyle alterations, is frequently contraindicated when there is evidence of liver or lung metastasis. Either of these metastases is readily diagnosed by noninvasive preoperative tests. Direct exploration at surgery is also necessary and very helpful, but that cannot replace the battery of indirect diagnostic tests termed the metastatic workup.

The testing inherent in a metastatic workup varies considerably, depending on the idiosyncrasies of the primary cancer. For example, most intestinal cancers typically metastasize first to regional lymph glands, then to liver and lung. Indirect laboratory studies are hard put to prove early lymphatic spread, but a minimum metastatic workup for colon or stomach cancer would include a chest X-ray and liver function blood studies. More sophisticated studies, such as magnetic resonance imaging (MRI), might follow if simpler studies are equivocal.

Prostate cancer has the unusual predilection to spread to bone, also lymph glands, liver, and lungs. Because of this, my metastatic workup included a chest X-ray, liver function blood studies, a prostatic acid phosphatase (PAP) blood test and a radioisotope bone scan.

Cancer metastasis to bone can sometimes produce pain indistinguishable from arthritis pain. For at least the last two years my "arthritis" had been increasingly active, especially in my neck, wrists, and hands. I've also had recurrent low back problems periodically that are typical of "acute facet syndrome." This is a common malady that causes severe low back pain, but is of no lasting clinical significance. Until recently, the only import in all that was a great excuse for why my golf game was deteriorating. Now, I had concern about what bad news my bone scan might announce. When you're having a run of bad luck, the mind really tends to run amok!

Although I had never undergone a radioisotope bone scan, I had used the procedure often in my clinical practice. I was very familiar with the indications and usefulness of the study. The end product looks like a picture of a miniature skeleton superimposed on transparent celluloid. A normal study shows a homogeneous bone pattern throughout. An abnormal scan may show areas of increased or decreased density over areas of diseased bone. A skilled radiologist can predict the cause of any bony abnormality.

Actually undergoing the bone scan proved to be an interesting experience. In preparation, a patient is asked to forego any liquids by mouth for several hours to become slightly dehydrated. Next, the technician asks the patient to empty the bladder (in privacy, of course). Then he or she injects a small dose of a radioactive isotope intravenously. The patient is asked to lie very still on an X-ray table on his back while the isotope scanner passes interminably slowly just above the body from head to foot. After it passes below the hands, which are placed at the sides—about twenty-five minutes into the procedure— the patient is allowed to scratch his nose, or whatever; but the lower body must remain completely motionless until the scanner passes below foot level—another twenty minutes or so. Then, after a brief time out, the process is repeated as the scanner passes posteriorly. Between passages, the technician asks that the patient again forcefully empty his bladder. This preoccupation with urination isn't just for the patient's comfort. Since the kidneys are actively excreting the radioactive isotope, a full bladder of isotope-containing urine will create a pelvic "hot spot." The hot spot can obstruct the view of part of the large pelvic bones, typical sites for some tumor metastases, including prostate cancer.

Knowing I was a physician, the technician allowed me to view my anterior scan film after she developed it and before proceeding to the posterior scan. It was normal to my inexpert eye, which relieved my anxiety considerably. But she didn't let me off the hook that easily. After completing the posterior scan, the technician left to develop the film. Upon her return she announced that she needed to take some supplemental scans of an area of my right chest. "I think it's just an artifact," she stated blandly.

After another thirty minutes of mind-torturing manipulation and technical maneuvering, she announced that we were finished. By that time I was a nervous wreck again. I convinced her that my sanity required that I meet the radiologist now to get his verdict. She and I took all the films, including my chest X-ray done earlier, to the radiologist's office in another part of the hospital. In my presence he studied all the films meticulously and tediously. Finally, he declared, "Everything looks okay to me." He didn't even comment on the "artifact," and I wasn't about to ask.

Later, I would learn that my liver function studies and PAP were normal, as I expected. Interpretation: As Dr. Williams had predicted, I had every indirect indication that my prostate cancer was small, well localized, and curable.

CHAPTER 6

Knowledge comes, but wisdom lingers.

—Alfred, Lord Tennyson

Dr. Williams had scheduled my next appointment for Monday, February 24. He wanted me to meet one of his new urological associates and have him examine me and review my case. Then, we three could discuss the findings of my metastatic workup and make concrete plans for my definitive treatment.

Dr. Williams' new partner was undoubtedly a very bright young urologist. It was obvious that he had an impressive grasp of urological knowledge and was very thorough, but his professional persona didn't favorably impress this former surgeon. To be specific, his digital rectal examination of my prostate was rough, prolonged, and hurt like hell. In my judgment, he definitely lacked the empathetic personal touch so important in the practice of the medical arts.

During my own clinical practice years, and as a teacher of surgery, I sometimes felt intellectually inferior to the brightest of my capable and learned staff of young university-trained surgeons. I noted, however, that many of them seemed too mechanical in their approach to patient care, which often offended my sensibilities. During my teaching rounds I had insisted that my students be "gentle doctors," whether performing an examination on an alert patient or doing an operation under anesthesia. I repeatedly stressed the fact that careful handling of living tissue during surgery would minimize cell injury and the development of many complications. Also, postoperative pain would be less severe. It was apparent to me then that some of my younger colleagues were not nearly so tuned in to the importance of this principle as I. They considered my fetish of gentle surgical technique as unnecessary and "old womanish."

Either I got through to Dr. Williams during his surgical training or he remembered my admonitions and treated me according to my teachings—I like to believe it was the former. His examinations were always deliberate and very gentle. Although his younger associate was obviously very sharp and knowledgeable, I wouldn't have allowed him to be my primary surgeon because of his roughness. I felt confident that he would be an able surgical assistant, consultant, and backup for Dr. Williams, however.

My inclination was to opt for my operation ASAP under the old surgical principle that the longer a known cancer was present in your body the greater the chance it might spread. Dr. Williams convinced me this wasn't important with prostate cancer. His thinking was influenced by the conviction that my tumor was an extremely early one (by all indications). Also, it is a fact that prostate cancer is typically very indolent and slow to metastasize.

We decided to schedule my surgery for Monday, March 16. In the interim, I would bank two units (500 cc each) of my own blood for the chance that I would need an intraoperative or postoperative transfusion. The second unit could not be collected until more than two weeks after the first had been drawn. In this era of autoimmune deficiency syndrome (AIDS), I needed little convincing that to delay surgery to have my own blood available for transfusion was wise and conservative.

By this time, as if my head wasn't already full of concerns, Joe had to give me something else to worry about. "I've avoided telling you this, Dr. Payne, but we need to do a cystoscopy and 'RU' before surgery," Dr. Williams said matter-of-factly. "We need to make sure there isn't any bladder pathology, and we have to know exactly where the ureters enter the bladder. And we also want to make sure there aren't any more stones in your kidneys." (I had passed two kidney stones in years past).

"RU" is medical shorthand for retrograde urogram. In this cystoscopic procedure, catheters are slipped into the ureters at their entrance to the bladder. Radiographic contrast material is injected retrograde into each kidney through the catheters while making an X-ray. Joe explained to me that the ureters may vary in their anatomical junction with the bladder, sometimes entering very close to the prostate. Careful preoperative definition of those anatomical relationships was necessary.

"And, of course, we can evaluate the inside of the bladder and the prostatic urethra to make sure there's nothing else there," the doctor added.

Great! I thought to myself. I was worried I wouldn't have anything else bad to prey on my mind for the next two weeks.

Beyond my naturally fatalistic concern about the possibility of finding another cancer in my bladder, or worse, in a kidney, my experience with the retrograde urogram was less than congenial. As a second-year medical student, I mysteriously developed acute pyelonephritis, an unusual kidney infection for a healthy, young adult male. A diagnostic RU made during my illness caused severe and unrelenting renal colic—a complication that lasted for over a week. It was so terribly painful at the time that I literally prayed to die. Dr. Williams was sure my bad experience represented faulty procedural technique and wouldn't happen again, but naturally I wasn't completely convinced.

Dr. Williams scheduled the cystoscopy and retrograde urogram Friday before my scheduled surgery—Friday the 13th!

Later that same afternoon I had my first unit of blood drawn for banking—essentially a pint. This was done at a local, freestanding blood bank in Austin that serves as the blood center for all local hospitals. As a destitute medical student I had sold my blood regularly to help feed my family, so this was no biggie for me.

The blood bank procedures hadn't changed much over the years, except that now, considerable emphasis was placed on HIV determination and AIDS detection. Some detection techniques were innovative, or even quirky, depending on your point of view. For example, I did a double-take when my female interviewer suddenly asked, "Have any of your male sex partners in the last two years tested positive for AIDS?"

"Hmm. Not that I know of," I answered, and was immediately embarrassed. What wrong message had I inadvertently thrown her about my straight-arrow, heterosexual lifestyle? She went on to the next question, an innocuous one, without missing a beat. What a strange new world we live in!

The blood drawing itself went without incident. About two weeks later I repeated the whole process to obtain and bank my second unit of blood. No problems or difficulties. So far, so good.

CHAPTER 7

I am always ready to learn, but I do not always like being taught.

—Winston Churchill

Friday, March 13, 1992, was an interesting day in my life. I dreaded the cystoscopy because it's a painful procedure in a male, even if done expertly. The unavoidable trauma to the urethra during the procedure causes burning on urination for at least the rest of the day. I feared the retrograde urogram even more.

My procedure was scheduled for 9:30 A.M. Linden accompanied me, and, in my anxiety, we left home much too early. When it became apparent that we were facing a sit in the doctor's waiting room of more than thirty minutes, we opted to take a time-killing drive in the south Austin rurals. The morning was fresh, quiet, and overcast. Everything I saw had an aura of newness and an intensity of color or motion. It's hard to explain, but it was one of those humdrum experiences that stands out in remembrance, probably because of anxiety and other intense emotions I was experiencing.

The procedure came off unpleasant, as predicted, but without complications. Dr. Williams worked fast, gently, and efficiently. He found no internal evidence of cancer. The ureterovesical junctions were in favorable positions anatomically, and my kidneys were normal bilaterally. I experienced no untoward aftereffects except the expected dysuria (burning on urination) for a day or so. Later, Dr. Williams confided that I had passed another of his personal tests of which I was unaware at the time.

"A lot of my patients talk a good game, Dr. Payne," said Joe, during an early postoperative visit, "but I wasn't sure what kind of patient you'd be until after that cystoscopy. I can almost always predict how to expect a patient to do after surgery by how they react to the 'cysto.' And after the way you handled that, I knew you'd do just fine." I couldn't wait to add that kudo to my résumé.

My hospital preadmission interview was scheduled with a beautiful telephone voice named Sherry Baker at 3:00 P.M. that same day at Austin's Seton Northwest Medical Center. When Linden and I arrived at the hospital, less than a mile from our home as the crow flies, we were escorted to the preadmission interview area. Nurse Sherry greeted us there. She was as pleasant and attractive as her telephone voice. After the obligatory questions about my address, age, religion, insurance coverage, etc., she asked about my past medical history and took a good review of medical systems. Then she gave me instructions about what time to present myself for surgery and what not to eat and drink before admission.

"Nothing by mouth after midnight, Dr. Payne. Nothing! No chewing gum, no coffee, no water, nothing! Any questions?" Her big, blue eyes frowned at me in emphatic seriousness.

After Sherry gave me some standard literature about the hospital and its policies, I handed her the forms confirming the availability of my banked blood. Then I presented her with a copy of my "living will" to include in my official hospital records. A few days earlier I had prepared and signed this legal document—a written directive that all measures to support life be ended if death is certain and imminent. Unheard of until recently, a living will has become increasingly well accepted. When properly executed and after appropriate discussion and agreement by one's family, such an instrument can convey peace of mind to everyone concerned. A patient and his or her loved ones understand and agree that dignified demise will be allowed when physicians agree that death is inevitable. Health care professionals appreciate their patients' rationality and forethought. More practically, it allows the medical team to be less concerned about the possible legal ramifications of their ethical and conscientious treatment decisions with respect to unforeseen catastrophic complications.

While preparing my living will, I also executed an

instrument that granted permission to allow harvest and transplantation of my viable organs in case of my death. Many otherwise healthy people's lives depend on the availability of a timely organ transplant, which is possible only when someone else dies. To me, it's illogical, perhaps immoral, to uselessly bury functional kidneys, hearts, and other organs when there exists such an overwhelming need for this "gift of life." Today, the ability to use transplanted organs is expanding rapidly to include livers and lungs, and even pancreatic tissue. Who knows what all will be possible in future years?

Ms. Baker neatly placed all my accumulated paperwork in a manila folder and stashed it away with a flourish. She had handled this part very professionally, and I was duly impressed. But the time had come to draw my preoperative blood sample, and her cool, professional demeanor crashed and burned. When the first needle-stick missed my vein and was nonproductive of blood, she became so distressed I thought she might cry.

"Oh, I knew this was going to happen when I learned I was going to have to preadmit a doctor!" she moaned. Until that time her veil of self-confidence was so opaque that I had had no idea she was so intimidated by such a pussycat as I. "Please, God," she murmured to the Almighty, "let me hit a vein on this next try!"

I did my fatherly best to reassure Nurse Sherry. I told her that after the diversity of probing I had endured so far it was virtually impossible for her to discomfit me with a little bloodletting setback. She seemed grateful for that. On the next try, she was successful.

Sherry wished me a successful operation and directed me to preoperative anesthesia. Linden and I proceeded to a small office off the surgical suite where the anesthesiologist doing preanesthesia checks for Monday's surgery met us and introduced himself. Dr. Counts was dressed in his surgical greens under a white doctor's coat— typical attire for anesthesia folk. I learned he was one of thirty-three members of the Capital Anesthesiology Association, Inc., several of whom were stationed at Seton Northwest Hospital. In Austin, I presumed that a thirty-three-member group probably had the anesthesia business pretty well monopolized.

Dr. Counts first reviewed my medical records. Next, he asked me about problems with previous anesthetics, my medication history, and history of any recent acute illness. Then, he did a brief physical examination with emphasis on my heart and lungs. Finally, he explained that on the morning of surgery one of his anesthesiologist colleagues would meet me, prepare me for surgery, and conduct my anesthesia during the operation. As Dr. Williams and I had discussed earlier regarding anesthesia expectations, Dr. Counts recommended a light endotracheal anesthesia. That would be supplemented by an epidural catheter for administration of pain-controlling drugs. This catheter, a tiny polyethylene tube, would be directed into my spinal canal's epidural space via a spinal needle. The catheter would be secured in position by tape before my anesthetic was begun, and connected to a computer-controlled infusion machine. My catheter would remain in place after surgery for several days to control postoperative pain. The infusion machine would be programmed to deliver a continuous flow of medication, but it could be overridden by the patient (me!) to provide more frequent amounts of painkiller—up to a preset safe-upper-limit amount.

The computerized technique of continuous drug administration via epidural catheter was a recent innovation for postoperative pain control. That technology was developed after my retirement from clinical surgery, and I had had no experience with it. I questioned to myself how necessary it would be for a tiger like me, but the principle was reassuring.

Earlier, when Dr. Williams and I had talked about the risks of surgery, I reiterated to him every surgeon's first concern when going under the knife: the qualifications of the attending anesthetist. Anesthesiologists are doctors of medicine who have undergone several years of postgraduate medical training in the specialty of anesthesiology. Well-trained anesthesiologists provide anesthesia to patients of all age groups undergoing any scale of surgery, from short and simple operations to the most difficult and complex.

This doctor monitors your physiology during the procedure and properly doses your system with variably poisonous drugs necessary for the proper conduction of anesthesia. While practicing his art, the anesthesiologist literally holds your life-support systems in his hands.

Certified registered nurse anesthetists (CRNA) are graduate nurses who have taken special training in anesthesiology. They have subsequently passed rigorous licensure testing that certifies their knowledge and skill as an anesthetist. Many, but not all, CRNAs work under the supervision of a physician anesthesiologist. Most are highly-skilled technicians who can provide quality anesthesia for most operative situations, but most CRNAs eschew very-high-risk surgery unless they are part of an anesthesiologist-CRNA team. The team approach to anesthesia is ideal in many situations.

"I'm not particularly concerned about what you're going to be doing inside my belly, Joe, but I want you to assure me that the guy passing my gas is topnotch, and superbly trained!" I insisted on that more than once.

Dr. Counts and I exchanged more pleasantries (we had both trained in military hospitals in San Antonio). Finally, he wished me good luck and promised he would relay my history to my likely anesthesiologist for Monday—a Dr. Malone.

When Linden and I finally left the hospital with admission paperwork in hand, we both felt reassured. For myself, I was very relieved that this tedious day was coming to a conclusion without my receiving additional bad news—for a change. For her, she had positive vibes about the hospital and the professional staff we had met. They would take good care of her life partner!

CHAPTER 8

The greatest thing in family life is to take a hint when a hint is intended–and not to take a hint when a hint isn't intended.

–Robert Frost

Never having faced major surgery of this magnitude before, and imbued with the fatalist attitude of a surgeon (soberly able to predict even the most remote potentially disastrous complications), I was a bit miffed at the cavalier attitude of my sons when I first notified them of my planned operation. I expected them to encircle the wagons psychologically and fly to their mother's side (really, my side) immediately. But neither expressed a serious interest in coming home for my surgery at first. Eventually, they realized I had been diagnosed with a potentially deadly condition and would undergo a serious operation having major implications for the present and future. Both eventually made the decision to come to Austin for my operation.

My older son, Frank, and his younger brother, Jimmy, are both excellent physical specimens of young American manhood. They're what Linden calls Irish twins—both born in the same calendar year, only ten and a half months apart. Both share an absolutely heartwarming love and respect for their mother, which they display frequently and often. Besides that single trait they're as different as night from day.

Frank is of average height, wiry in build, quite handsome physically, but possesses little academic talent. As a star athlete in high school he was extremely popular with his teammates, other friends, and young women; but he barely managed to graduate, and was a complete bust in every after-high-school educational endeavor he attempted. He failed all of his courses in his two years of college majoring in "campusology." Frank busted out of the Air Force academically, and later the Marines—though never due to misconduct. Later, he survived an ill-conceived marriage that lasted less than two years (one year longer than I had predicted). Thankfully, the marriage did not produce any offspring. Subsequently, Frank successfully trained to become a manager of a Montana rental car agency and continues to do well. His mom and I have been quite proud of his late-developing maturity and his ability to pull himself up by his bootstraps to turn his life around.

Jimmy is a gentle giant who was frequently overshadowed in high school by his older brother's more sensational exploits. At 6 feet 2 inches and 240 pounds of pure muscle, he towered over Frank, but was slower and less agile. Jimmy did well academically in high school. He also excelled in sports, but in a less glamorous role. He quietly earned an appointment to the Air Force Academy. There, he was successful academically, played varsity football, qualified for flight training, and became an Air Force fighter pilot after graduation. While growing up he continually amazed his mother and me with the depth of judgment and maturity he exhibited, in contrast to his brother. We used to describe Jimmy as "age seventeen going on thirty-five."

My only daughter, Valerie, is six years older than Frank, married, the mother of four young children, and a professional photographer in Sacramento, California. Although Val and Linden have established a warm mother-daughter relationship, she and I have not communicated very effectively for several years. The possibility of Val's coming to Austin for my surgery was never a consideration.

I felt strongly about the boys being present for my operation since I wasn't convinced I would survive the anesthesia (I still wasn't particularly worried about surviving the surgery). That having been decided, Jimmy arrived from his duty station in South Carolina that Friday evening. Frank was due to arrive from his home in Montana the next afternoon.

Linden and I had planned a trip Saturday morning to a shopping mall to buy me a couple of pairs of good pajamas and a robe. I hadn't worn pajamas since the first fifteen minutes of my wedding night in 1962 and didn't own either pajamas or a robe. Linden was not about to let me wear my undershorts in the hospital, and I didn't cotton to the standard tie-in-the-back hospital gown. I had decided to go first class and not let expense be a factor in the purchase of my hospital wardrobe. If I lived to wear new pajamas in the hospital, they were definitely going to be classy and expensive.

We eventually shopped at three different men's apparel shops before we found the pajamas and a colorful silk robe to my liking. With my family now in tow and my hospital wardrobe intact, I was ready for my hospital experience, both mentally and sartorially.

Although I was completely self-absorbed with my upcoming trial by fire, it was obvious my sons weren't taking things quite so seriously. Before Jimmy went to the airport Saturday afternoon to meet Frank's incoming plane, he searched out a professional costume shop. He rented a funky, hippie wig, fake moustache and beard, and donned a long overcoat. He must have looked about as grungy and unkempt as imaginable. He stumbled all over Frank at the arrival gate, apparently played the confrontation scene to the hilt, and both almost got arrested by airport security police. They told Linden and me the story with verve and imagination, and both thought it was a great joke.

That night we had a fine dinner at Jeffrey's, my very favorite restaurant in Austin and the world. The establishment did their culinary magic marvelously, as expected. We all agreed the dinner was delicious, the wine was perfect, and the company was warm and supportive of Dad. I slept well that night in Linden's loving arms.

I continued to subconsciously deny any sickness or human weakness by running two and a half miles Sunday morning (as I had Saturday, also). I can't remember exactly what my thoughts were during those preoperative, early morning jogs. I probably felt that proving my stamina by strenuous, physical activity might somehow be redeeming to this breakdown of physical perfection I knew was going on inside my body. After a long, soothing soak in the spa after my workout, I showered with Betadine antiseptic soap I had previously purchased at a drugstore. This was good surgical practice, and I insisted that my patients use an antiseptic soap for their bath the day before surgery. It couldn't hurt, I figured.

We all felt edgy and nervous most of that Sunday during the day. In the evening, though, I had decided to have a charcoal-grilled porterhouse steak for my "last supper." One of my greatest talents is my skill in preparing steaks grilled to gastronomic perfection. All Payne family members agree on that truth. I figured that this evening was not the time to be concerned about cholesterol, saturated fats, and whatnot. To complement my steak I opened a precious bottle of my Heitz Cellars' Cabernet Sauvignon, Martha's Vineyard, vintage 1967, which I had been hoarding since the early '70s. While decanting it carefully and skillfully I gave thanks that my wife and sons didn't care for wine, leaving more for my enjoyment alone. The dinner was outstanding even by my own standards.

Five o'clock on the morning of Monday, March 16, 1992, would come quickly, early, dark, dreary, and, to me, ominous and frightening.

CHAPTER 9

The natural role of twentieth-century man is anxiety.

—Norman Mailer

The alarm on the radio at the head of my bed went off at 5:00 A.M. and I awoke with a start. I must have slept some that last night before my surgery, although it's hard to believe. Naturally, Linden had efficiently packed all my personal and bathroom gear for the hospital before we retired for the night, so there wasn't much preparation necessary. I wasn't supposed to eat or drink anything that morning—not even a cup of black coffee—so I didn't. No way would I dare let myself contribute any personal blame for whatever horrible anesthetic complication I might have in the next few hours.

Frank and Jimmy were up and about when Linden and I emerged from the master bedroom. None of us were in the mood for small talk. Although Linden is the only "morning person" in the family, she was as subdued and noncommunicative as the rest of us. It was a strange and artificial atmosphere that early morning of March 16.

As with every family outing since my children were born, I was still the daddy, not yet the patient, so I drove us the short distance to Seton Northwest Medical Center. It was still pitch dark outside—a clear, starry night, and unseasonably warm. After parking and locking the car in the eerily illuminated, almost empty parking area, we walked together into the hospital's brightly lit main corridor. The hallway was deserted at that early hour. All this brightness seemed somehow offensive to me. It didn't properly match the still very dark night—a night as dark and somber as my mood.

A middle-aged couple and their frightened-looking

teenage daughter shared the elevator with us to the surgical suite. I learned later the young lady was scheduled for a knee operation that morning. None of us spoke during the short elevator trip.

Within the surgical suite the activity level was much greater. A dozen or more people in surgical greens were moving about smartly in all directions, appearing and disappearing from various doorways and curtained cubicles. When we arrived, a male orderly led us to a cubicle that enclosed a very uncomfortable, pillowless gurney covered by a tightly drawn, wrinkle-free white sheet. There was a heavy steel step-up on the floor, and not much else. The orderly asked me to disrobe, don a hospital gown—the kind that are open in the rear—and hop aboard the gurney. Before waltzing out through the closed curtains he perfunctorily plopped down a fresh, white, folded sheet on the gurney. Presumably, I was to hide under it after I was properly gowned and downed.

Despite the hustle and bustle of the surgical suite personnel, it turned out that my elevator mate and I were the only two patients being prepared for early surgery. A slow operating morning today, perhaps. It occurred to me then that I had always tried to avoid scheduling my own major surgeries for Monday mornings. I could usually prepare myself to do a big operation, but other personnel would be likely to have "blue Monday" attitude. Not a good thing, because surgery is very much a team endeavor.

Linden and my sons joined me in my cubicle after I had removed my street clothes and transmuted from a human being into a patient. As I laid uncomfortably on the gurney under the bright lights of the surgery suite with my family hovering, I felt very out of place in this surrealistic environment. Shortly, a professional-appearing male technician entered our world and very coolly and adroitly placed an intravenous line into an accessible vein in my left hand. He secured the catheter in place with transparent tape and started a slow infusion of electrolyte solution. My anesthesiologist-of-the-day then came in, politely introduced himself, and reviewed my anesthesia and medical history again, point by point. He explained that he would soon give me a medication intravenously to allay anxiety and make me drowsy. Because of my general good health, he decided I didn't need an electrocardiogram (EKG), a study that Dr. Williams had previously ordered to be accomplished before my surgery. I vaguely remembered a small flap taking place around me regarding the EKG decision, then a technician hooking me up to the EKG apparatus.

Then, suddenly and without warning: BAROOM! CLANG! BAROOM! I was hearing loud, tinny, uncoordinated musical sounds like the background musical sound effects on "Law and Order," the TV show. I was rudely shocked into consciousness and jostled around as if I were in an out-of-control raft on a stormy sea. Groggily, I became more aware of this flurry of activity all around me by many green-gowned hospital personnel—male and female. Then I realized what was happening. They were shifting me into my hospital room bed from an operating room recovery bed. All sorts of tubes, bandages, bloody fluid-filled plastic bags, and various other paraphernalia were protruding from various sites on my body. The various foreign materials were swinging back and forth, pulling at my belly, my penis, my arm, and many other places. I didn't seem to hurt anywhere exactly, although the jostling was distinctly unpleasant. It seemed like Mardi Gras was happening in my room, and my badly violated carcass wasn't in the mood to party. I tried to be helpful, I thought, but in my present frame of mind, I didn't want to be bothered.

Soon, enough cobwebs cleared from my mind that I realized my operation had taken place. It was over. I had survived my surgery. I was alive. What a surprise! Now, I thought, I'll have to hunker down and go through my postoperative recovery.

Just as I was coming to this realization, Dr. Williams breezed into the room, maneuvered himself through the herd of busy bodies and hands, leaned over my bed, and poked his grinning face in front of mine. "You did fine, Dr. Payne!" he barked cheerfully, as if I were hard of hearing. "Your operation is over! The lymph nodes were negative, and we were able to do the radical prostatectomy! Everything went real, real well! Do you understand?" I understood perfectly, but I couldn't have cared less right then. I probably nodded my head.

Dr. Williams quickly inspected various hoses and bags, made a few quick, minor alterations of tubes and drains, and breezed out as quickly as he had appeared. In the background toward the foot of my bed, I saw Linden and my sons standing rigid and looking awkward amongst the flurry of activity that was now slowing. One by one or two, the hospital folk began to disperse, some wheeling out equipment on a gurney or stand, others carrying out smaller bundles. Others just disappeared into the corridor as they finished their tasks. Finally, after a short while, it was just my family and me. Linden searched anxiously for something to do that she hoped would make me more comfortable. Frank and Jimmy appeared distinctly ill at ease, and notably green around the gills. I was too mentally discomfited to go soundly to sleep, but was unable to fully shake my cerebral fuzziness. I found myself constantly dozing off and snapping back awake with a start.

During an episode of consciousness, I became aware of many strange, unattractive, and distinctly cumbersome medical supplies plugged into my body in various places. These made snuggling into a comfortable bed position impossible. I was immediately thankful that I had no nasogastric tube or other oral or nasal catheters. A Foley urinary catheter had been placed into my bladder through my penis, however. The mulatto brown rubber tube was securely taped to the upper part of my right thigh. It was attached by clear plastic tubing to a large plastic bag hanging off the right side of my bed. The bag contained roughly 300 cc of grossly bloody urine that was already becoming clear yellow in the upper tubing. I was mildly surprised that the catheter wasn't grossly uncomfortable. That perception would soon change.

Every half-minute or so, a whirring sound like a tiny fan came on, accompanied by a strange massaging action in my legs. The sensation began just above my ankles and migrated progressively upward into my midthighs over a period of a few seconds. This would startle or sometimes awaken me, but it wasn't painful or uncomfortable. In due time I learned that this apparatus was the state of the art technology for preventing venous stasis and possible pulmonary thromboembolism, replacing the Jobst dynamic elastic vascular stockings of my surgical era.

I felt a soft lump taped to my low back the size of a softball. Coming out of the taped lump and traversing up and over my left shoulder was a tiny polyethylene catheter. The catheter was attached to a metal rectangular box clamped to an intravenous fluid (IV) pole on the left side of my bed. The metal box had a gauge and several small knobs, and a hand-held control device resembling a nurse's call button that was strategically placed out of my reach. This little machine got much attention from the nursing personnel traipsing in and out. During my second postoperative day, when I was alert enough to ask, I learned that this was the computerized patient-controlled analgesia, or PCA. By using this, I could push a button to inject additional pain-relieving narcotic medication into the epidural space of my spine. There were some limitations with it, but I would learn about those later. During my first several postoperative hours I was not allowed to independently operate the PCA; but, in truth, I didn't need anything beyond what the anesthesiologist had programmed into the computer to be given automatically.

The most disquieting new items of apparel I had acquired were two suction drains attached to polyethylene catheters protruding from the skin of either side of my pelvis just above my groin. Each was held in place by a dressing loosely taped over my lower abdomen and connected to clear plastic bulbs, roughly the size and shape of hand grenades. Both were partially filled with bloody fluid. These were Jackson-Pratt drains. They were ingeniously designed little suction catheters. They could be emptied, compressed manually, then sealed at one end to create a vacuum suction for the tube attached to their opposite ends. Later, I learned that the tubes were placed deep into my pelvic retroperitoneal space. They were brought to the outside through small stab incisions just in front of my iliac crests bilaterally. When Dr. Williams changed their overlying dressings I was impressed that the exit sites were fashioned so bilaterally symmetrical.

These J-P drains, although functionally efficient, were the most cumbersome part of my new postoperative attire. I would eventually remember them with as much, or more, distaste as I had for my Foley catheter.

Finally, a loose gauze bandage covered my operative incision. I couldn't see it because of the dressing, but I was acutely aware of its presence, nonetheless. The incision extended from my belly button almost to the base of my penis, which now lay tiny and flaccid between my legs. It was skewered on an enormous rubber tube exiting the meatus. The operative incision, although not painful, was readily defined by an area of dull-sharp discomfort that always remained well within my tolerance.

So here I am. What now? I asked myself. As the next several hours of the day of surgery passed and evening faded into night, I dozed and roused. Usually, I was awakened when a nurse or aide came to empty, add, or measure; or when Linden stirred from her makeshift sleeping pad in a corner of my room. My lover and life partner, herself a registered nurse, was not ready to entrust my care on my first postoperative night to the mercy of untested health care professionals.

Seton Northwest Medical Center was a new hospital and was the epitome of the modern trend of medical facilities—all rooms were private; that is, one bed to a room. Not having to abide a stranger roommate (and his family) observing my misery and lost personal dignity was a blessing difficult to fully appreciate unless you've experienced it the other way. I had. But most important to my peace of mind during those early and frightening postoperative hours was having Linden able to stay with me in my room. I couldn't think clearly most of that first postoperative night and frequently would be awakened or startled into consciousness. Each time this happened I would see Linden and be reassured. Once, before drifting back into drug-induced, restless sleep, I decided firmly that since I had survived the surgery, and since my recovery was that important to Linden, I might as well by God go all the way and get well!

CHAPTER 10

Where everything is bad it must be good to know the worst.

—Francis H. Bradley

In my own surgical practice over the years, I observed that the day following surgery, called the first postoperative day, was the most uncomfortable time in a normal recovery period. I always forewarned my patients about this because they instinctively expected to feel as chipper on the first postoperative day as they did immediately after operation. Remembering this phenomenon I knew I would feel lousy Tuesday, March 17, my first postoperative day. I wasn't disappointed.

As dawn approached and the nursing day crew began to circulate, I awoke from a fitful sleep and tried to orient myself to the new day. I soon noticed that my soft palate and uvula had become very swollen and tender overnight. (The uvula is the tear-shaped soft tissue protrusion that hangs down from the soft palate in the back of the throat.) Although this was uncomfortable and annoying, my experience was that the problem was temporary and self-limited. I recalled several similar episodes of that syndrome occurring in my youth, presumably caused from mouth-breathing while in a deep sleep following intemperate alcohol use.

As the morning passed, I tried to ignore my constant frog-in-the-throat feeling. I ambulated around the hallway without much difficulty and was experiencing no nausea or significant pain. Dr. Williams visited on his morning rounds and removed my dressing, allowing my first peek at my operative incision. While he dressed my wounds and adjusted my drains, he talked to me again about how well the operation went and his considerable optimism about my findings at surgery. Apparently, the operation was without incident, my anatomy was easy to work with, bleeding was minimal, and there was no visible gross tumor anywhere. He saved the nerves necessary for erections, and expressed the opinion that I should regain potency in six to eighteen months (but no guarantees!).

As Dr. Williams emptied my J-P drains, he explained that these catheters were placed in the retroperitoneal space to evacuate any bleeding or leak from the bladder-urethra anastomosis and to prevent lymphocele formation. Whenever lymphatic tissue is excised, it is virtually impossible to ligate all the tiny lymphatic vessels; therefore, it is necessary to drain the area of leaking lymph fluid until the drainage stops, usually in a few days. Otherwise, a collection of the lymph, a lymphocele, could form and become infected or require surgery for drainage.

When the daily drainage output from either J-P drain decreased below a minimum amount, he would remove that drain. The opposite side tube and drain would be ready for removal a week later, probably. The doctor explained that I would empty and recharge the drains myself at home after I left the hospital, presumably in four days.

My incision was just as I had pictured it. It extended from just below my umbilicus almost to the base of my penis. The skin edges were approximated with closely placed metal skin clips. There was no bleeding, ecchymosis (bruising) or other obvious problem. It was a very clean and neat incision. I was impressed!

Dr. Williams asked me if the leg massagers "bugged" me (they didn't, but apparently the sound and vibrations bother many patients). He explained that removing the pelvic lymph nodes interrupted the lymphatic vessels of the pelvis that drain the lower extremities. Because of that, leg edema (swelling) can quickly develop from prolonged inactivity, such as bed rest. Also, venous stasis in the legs can lead to phlebothrombosis, a serious complication that permanently damages the blood circulation to the lower extremities. It can also lead to pulmonary embolism, where a blood clot in a leg vein breaks off and travels through the blood stream to the lungs. Pulmonary embolism is a dreaded, often fatal, postoperative complication to be avoided at all costs. Dr. Williams routinely used this leg massage therapy after prostate cancer surgery to increase venous blood flow and interrupt the chain of events that lead to these complications.

To get back to my throat problem: After the activities of the previous night and morning, Linden needed to get some rest at home. Jimmy elected to take her home and planned to run some personal errands. Frank was drafted to stay with me at the hospital. I was testy and uncomfortable, and Frank was out of his element trying to be a care-giver to a sick patient. He tried hard, but required lots of breaks to the cafeteria or elsewhere.

While lying in bed I could tell that my throat swelling wasn't lessening, and it was becoming harder to breathe easily. Although I thought it was getting worse, I wasn't certain whether that was real or my active imagination. To make matters worse, an older couple who had been our neighbors in our previous home came to visit. When they entered my room Frank disappeared, leaving me to entertain them alone. The old gentleman was surprised I wasn't as spry as he had been after his transurethral resection, an operation to relieve urinary obstruction due to prostatic hyperplasia. (I wasn't motivated to explain to him that a TUR was immeasurably different from prostate cancer surgery). My general discomfort, combined with anxiety about my respiratory difficulty, made it impossible for me to be a genial host. When my visitors finally left after getting the message that their visit was too early to be therapeutic, I asked the nurse to have someone inspect my throat. An on-call anesthesiologist came by shortly and was impressed with the degree of edema in my soft palate. He made the immediate decision to have me taken back to the surgical recovery room for close observation and treatment.

During the next six hours I was treated with oxygen mist by face mask and systemic steroids by injection to try to reduce the pharyngeal edema. As the hours passed without apparent improvement by my appraisal, I became more and more terrified. My imagination ran wild with visions of worsening laryngeal edema, the need for endotracheal intubation, perhaps surgical tracheostomy, or worse.

As mentioned earlier, the problem with being a doctor patient, especially for a surgeon, is that you know all the complications that can occur and their worst possible outcomes. For example, part of my treatment for my throat edema was racemic epinephrine solution in the oxygen mist. A physiological side effect of epinephrine is elevated blood pressure. Naturally, I made the nurse tell me what my blood pressure was every time she took it. And, not surprising, it was higher than the previous reading every time. Having nothing better to do, I systematically visualized all the symptoms and complications of malignant hypertension, including seizures, stroke, myocardial infarction, etc. Surprise! Surprise! My blood pressure continued to climb.

After several hours my throat swelling finally began to improve ever so slightly. By then, I had decided I had rather die in my room than suffer the pangs of misery my mind was conjuring up in that surgical recovery room. With considerable effort I called up enough professional reserve to convince the anesthesiologist treating me that I could return to the ward. Two or three sublingual Procardia tablets reduced my high blood pressure to a reasonable level, and he agreed to send me back to my room. I did fine. By the next morning the swelling had completely subsided. Now I could enjoy worrying about the common surgical complications that typically occur on the second through seventh postoperative day. These include thrombophlebitis (blood clot and inflammation of a vein), abscess formation, wound dehiscence (the parting of the sutured lips of an incision), pneumonia, and other gory things.

CHAPTER 11

There is no failure except in no longer trying. There is no defeat except from within, no really insurmountable barrier save our own inherent weakness of purpose.

—Kin Hubbard

In the hospital I was a good patient by anyone's standards. I required only occasional supplemental pain medication and could cough and breathe deeply without difficulty—patient characteristics guaranteed to please nurses. It was a surprise that I had so little incision discomfort, even with coughing or straining. In my practice, abdominal surgery patients usually complained of significant incision pain while straining to cough—and an unguarded sneeze was torture. Since my discomfort was so minimal, I decided my pain threshold must be great. I had failed to consider the effect of my epidural catheter and PCA, with its continuous infusion of pain medication. My anesthesiologist brought this to my attention when I bragged about my stoicism. He assured me it would be unwise to remove my epidural catheter on the second postoperative day. I had the good sense not to challenge that opinion.

By now I was becoming acutely aware of my indwelling Foley catheter. Not only did it pull in all the wrong places with every movement I made, but the irritation of the tubing was causing marked soft tissue swelling of my prepuce. It looked horrible—like a pink stalk of broccoli growing around a brown rubber tube. Dr. Williams was unconcerned with the swelling. He reassured me that the edema was transitory and less severe than average.

Resplendent in my rich-looking royal blue pajamas

under a silk, wine-colored robe, I began to walk the halls incessantly. The Foley catheter and its accouterments weren't the only hindrances to my mobility. I also had my intravenous fluids on an IV pole on rollers to drag along. My Jackson-Pratt drain bulbs would bob up and down as I walked. In my colorful garb, I must have looked like a Mardi Gras float as I paraded up and down the corridors.

The first purpose of my desire for early and frequent ambulation was to preclude the possibility of venous stasis problems in my legs. Also, I wanted to try to get intestinal gas moving. A significant side effect of abdominal surgery is the inevitable development of intestinal atony (paralysis or inactivity) for various periods of time postoperatively. The degree of atony depends mainly on the magnitude of the operation. Atony is likely to be more severe and prolonged if the surgery is intraperitoneal; that is, within the abdominal cavity. This is especially true in an operation involving the bowel, such as a gastrectomy, colectomy, or even appendectomy. For a retroperitoneal procedure such as I had—one that doesn't actually violate the abdominal cavity—the period of bowel paresis is usually short. Return of function is determined by such mundane signs as intestinal rumbling and, more important, passing flatus. Most intestinal gas passed as flatus is previously swallowed air; therefore, lack of gas passage can't be blamed on diet restriction. The best way to get gas to pass is by being active, such as by walking. Active ambulation induces functional and productive peristalsis. Burping or belching doesn't count as a favorable sign of bowel activity. In fact, eructation and/or actual vomiting are bad signs, indicative that the intestinal tract is unable to move things along normally. In some major abdominal surgery, intestinal atony is such a common occurrence that a tube is routinely placed into the stomach by nasogastric passage and connected to gentle suction. Swallowed air and gastric secretions are then aspirated via the tube until physiological intestinal action resumes.

I was pleased that I didn't need nasogastric suction because it is unpleasant to have a stomach tube protruding from a nostril. This also inhibits deep breathing and increases the risk of pulmonary complications, such as pneumonia and atelectasis (collapse of lung tissue). But the only thing worse than having a nasogastric tube is to need one therapeutically and not have it. In that situation a patient must contend with the abdominal muscles straining to retch and vomit against a new and tender abdominal incision. The addition of gastric distention from swallowed air and secretions that aren't moving as they should combine for a terrible misery. These problems can lead to potentially fatal complications in a worst-case scenario. Thoughtful surgeons must use excellent judgment to decide upon the use of nasogastric intubation.

When I hadn't yet passed gas after my first postoperative day and had experienced minimal borborygmi (stomach "growling"), I decided that I would continue to walk the halls until I did so. I surely didn't want to have a stomach tube placed while I was awake and alert. I had had that done once as a medical student, and once was plenty. Sure enough, during the late morning of the second postoperative day, my ambulation efforts were rewarded. I passed considerable prolonged, high-pitched crepitus that not only relieved my increasing anxiety, but filled me with pride of authorship. The nurses rewarded me with a clear liquid diet. After that I passed even more gas.

A not uncommon complication of abdominal surgery, especially urologic surgery, is the development of an abdominal or retroperitoneal abscess. Since my surgery was totally retroperitoneal (behind the membrane that lines the cavity of the abdomen), I was at some risk for a retroperitoneal abscess. Such an abscess usually develops from infection of a collection of blood oozing into the operative area postoperatively. Such oozing may occur for several days after operation and is virtually impossible to prevent, although the volume is seldom significant from a hemodynamic standpoint. It is most important to evacuate any ooze as it occurs to prevent this very dangerous and life-threatening complication. The purpose of my Jackson-Pratt drains, plastic catheters placed deep into the pelvic retroperitoneum bilaterally, was to affect this drainage. Nurses would empty the accumulated fluid from the J–P drains thrice daily and carefully record the volume collected from each side. The drainage approximated 100–150 cc from each on the first day after surgery, but it decreased each consecutive day, as expected. By the fourth postoperative day, the right drain had practically ceased to produce at all. The left side was still draining over 60 cc per day, however—the magic number considered "dry" by surgical standards.

Dr. Williams had promised to remove the right drain before my discharge from the hospital. I looked forward to this because the drains were really bothersome and cumbersome little devils. They would constantly bob up and down, bouncing off my tender incision, or pull at the skin suture holding the plastic tubing in place. I reasoned that removal of one would at least lessen the irritation by half.

I thought little about the removal procedure, but this turned out to be an unusual and uncomfortable event, the likes of which I had never experienced. Although there was no pain as usually interpreted, the sensual feel of a tube with multiple suction holes being forcibly extracted from the depths of a body cavity was shocking. It was also fleetingly nauseating and distinctly unpleasant. My reaction was minimal, which again impressed Dr. Williams, but my first thought later was that I had to go through that same trick again in a few days. Knowing how it would feel, would I be such a tough guy the next time? By the morning of my fourth postoperative day, Friday, March 20, I was ambulating well and eating a regular diet. I was experiencing no discomfort except the irritation of my Foley catheter and the remaining J-P drain. The swelling and edema of my penis foreskin thankfully had resolved nicely. Earlier, an anesthesiologist visited to follow up on my throat problem and to remove my epidural catheter, which turned out to be a simple procedure.

Despite my worst fears everything was going very well. I was ready to continue my convalescence at home.

CHAPTER 12

What we anticipate seldom occurs; what we least expect generally happens.

—Benjamin Disraeli

The day for my discharge having finally dawned, a nurse had placed my inpatient chart on the night table beside my bed, anticipating that Dr. Williams would sign my discharge order when he visited. Being alone in my room I picked up the chart, lifted the metal chart cover and discovered that the top page was my final pathology report. It's impossible to describe the panorama of emotions I experienced over the next several minutes as I read the report, first scanning it for the summary, then perusing it for detail.

The first page of the four-page report described only the pathologist's methodology for fixing the tissue and preparing it for examination microscopically. He followed the standard procedure: Small bits of tissue cut from strategic sites on the surgical specimen were placed in small metal cassettes and "fixed" in formalin solution. The morsels of tissue were then transferred to hot, liquid paraffin. The paraffin was allowed to cool, producing wax blocks approximately one-half inch square with the tissue in the center. Using a microtome, the paraffin blocks were shaved into thin slices onto microscope slides and stained with special dyes. The stained and dried slides were ready for examination under a microscope.

I quickly turned to page two. At midpage a paragraph began "MICROSCOPIC:". I read quickly, "No metastatic carcinoma in the lymph nodes harvested." So far, so good, and as I expected. The next sentence paragraph hit me like the proverbial ton of bricks: "Right vas deferens and seminal vesicle: Infiltrating adenocarcinoma present." I swallowed hard and, I think, began to shake a little as the impact of those nine words sunk in. Despite what the rest of the report would say, this short statement had transformed my completely curable, stage A, minimal cancer into a stage C, life-threatening cancer that may be incurable. And from now on, whatever else transpires, I will be inevitably at risk of dying from metastatic prostate cancer. At best, again based on that one line of the pathologist's report, I will face years of follow-up tests, each time having to sweat out the results. Forever, I'll wonder whether every arthritic pain is a bone metastasis of prostate cancer; every sickness, a cancer recurrence or spread.

There was even more bad news. The pathologist described an obviously aggressive tumor that was present in both lobes of the prostate. It extended to several margins of the surgical excision. The distal prostatic urethra showed tumor cells present. And there was perineural tumor invasion—a sign that cancer already may have been disseminated by the blood stream.

I read and reread the report until I realized I was no longer absorbing information, but was mentally trying to change the obvious truth of the data in my mind. It wasn't working. There was no way to rationally deny the hard truth. I finally closed the metal chart cover and sank dejectedly back into my pillow. There was nothing I could do.

Soon, Dr. Williams arrived to do my discharge paperwork. He opened the chart and began reading the pathology report, which was still the top document. The doctor wasn't aware I had already read it. At first he chatted with me lightly as he read, but as the impact of the report dawned on him, he soon fell silent. Dr. Williams read intently as had I, himself having difficulty absorbing the complicated descriptions completely; but undoubtedly understanding the impact of the obvious. Finally, he spoke. "Jim, your path report is here, and it's really not what we expected," he began. I would have liked to have helped him out by saying something glib, but I didn't know how. He continued, "There's really a lot more tumor present than we thought." Dr. Williams went on to discuss what the report said and what I already knew. I let him talk on, hoping he could somehow minimize the importance of the cold, descriptive truth in some way. Naturally, he couldn't.

There are many ways clinicians and pathologists stage cancer to attempt to predict the curability (or lethality) of the tumor, depending on several factors, including the tumor site and type. One of the simplest and most frequently used is the clinical/pathologic staging of A, B, C, and D. Clinical stage refers to the characteristics of the tumor as defined by the clinician on examination or at surgery. This is obviously gross and imperfect, but useful in planning treatment, and reasonably accurate. Pathological stage refers to the findings on examination of the tumor and surrounding tissue both grossly and microscopically by a pathologist after surgery. The pathologic stage is invariably definitive and accurate in almost all cases since the pathologist can take all the time and effort necessary to study the tissue. The tumor can literally be examined cell by cell.

In prostate cancer, stage A refers to cancers that are small and completely localized to the prostate gland. Stage B indicates localized spread within the gland, but still completely contained and not extending to the periphery. In stage C there is local spread to adjacent organs. Stage D1 indicates spread to contiguous lymph nodes. Stage D2 means the tumor has metastasized to one or more distant sites.

Obviously, stage A cancer has the best prognosis, and usually is considered highly curable. Stage B is almost as favorable for cure, but not quite. The percentages for complete cure decreases considerably with stage C tumors. They always carry the potential for recurrence and/or metastasis whatever the type and quality of treatment. Stage D suggests a grim prognosis almost invariably.

The specific percentages associated with cure rate in each stage vary with the type of cancer and its organ of origin, but the relationship of curability between the four stages generally remains constant. In prostate cancer, spread to a seminal vesicle is considered spread to a separate, adjacent organ and is, by definition, stage C.

Pathologists also use the Gleason histological grading to predict the relative aggressiveness of a prostate cancer.

This is the sum of the two most prevalent histologic patterns of the tumor added together. Prostatic malignancies are usually slowgrowing tumors. In very elderly men with a prostate cancer of low Gleason score, say Gleason 3–4, many clinicians feel that radical surgery may be more dangerous to the patient than the tumor itself. Use of the Gleason grading system by the pathologist ranks the tumor cells that make up the cancer from well differentiated (Gleason grade 2–5) to highly undifferentiated (Gleason grade 8–10). The well-differentiated prostate cancer can be predicted to be even slower-growing and nonaggressive in its clinical behavior. The highly undifferentiated cancer cells found in a Gleason grade 8, 9, or 10 may grow rapidly and be very active in terms of recurrence and metastasis. Moderately differentiated cell types in a Gleason grade 6–7 tend to behave somewhere between these extremes.

Pathologists will give a prostate cancer a Gleason grade that represents characteristic tumor cells in at least two areas of the cancer because each prostate cancer usually has cells that vary in maturity, or degree of differentiation, from site to site within the substance of the tumor. The Gleason score grades areas that represent the most-differentiated cancer cells and those areas where tumor cells are least differentiated. For example, a Gleason grade 5–6 would suggest a tumor consisting of cells of a slightly varying degree of moderate differentiation. This tumor would be potentially less aggressive than a Gleason grade 8–9, containing cells that were more bizarre in their microscopic appearance—less differentiated. The pathologist characterized my tumor cells as Gleason grade 6–7, moderately differentiated, nevertheless a potentially dangerous cancer. It could have been better, but then it could have been worse.

In days to follow, my reading would teach me that fully 40 percent of clinical stage A prostate cancers, meaning what is found by clinical examination before definitive surgery, turn out to be pathological stage C, as mine had.

"My main fear before your operation, Jim," Dr.

Williams continued, "was that I'd have to tell you the pathologist could not find any cancer in the specimen, and have you wondering whether I'd done this big operation on you for nothing. I never expected this," he said, gesturing to the chart and shaking his head slowly from side to side. Had I not been a physician, he might have resorted to all sorts of verbal gymnastics to soften this severe blow. I know. I've done it often—and without apology. But he knew I understood. And he knew it was futile for him to be anything less than straightforward with me.

We didn't talk much more, but shortly after that I was officially discharged from the hospital. Linden was cheerful and supportive and glad to be taking her honey home in one piece, more or less. I had yet to tell her about my pathology report. That could wait. It wasn't going to change, and I wasn't going to metastasize to death on the short ride home.

CHAPTER 13

The best way out is always through.

—Robert Frost

When Linden left the ward to bring our car to the hospital entrance, I collected all my connections and accouterments into a compact parcel in preparation for my eminent departure. My physical baggage included a low midline abdominal incision and attached metal skin clips, a Foley urinary catheter hooked up to a plastic leg bag (that was beginning to be a real bother), the Jackson-Pratt drain in my left lower abdomen, and a thick dressing on my low back where the epidural catheter had lived. I was weak and tired, emotionally drained, and had lost ten pounds in the last five days. I was experiencing no consistent pain, but had lots of areas of discomfort and irritation.

Knowing hospital rules, I settled myself into the wheelchair that had been mobilized for me. I then allowed myself to be ferried to the hospital entrance by a kindly, talkative, hospital volunteer lady. She was quite elderly, but surprisingly spry, so we moved along smartly. Without much ado, I transitioned from the wheelchair to the car seat without difficulty. Soon Linden and I were driving safely homeward. Physically, I was doing quite well, but I didn't realize how close I was to the edge, emotionally.

After settling in at home, I told Linden and Jimmy about the pathology report, its content, and my discussion with Dr. Williams. It was an emotional moment because I couldn't minimize my chagrin and disappointment, and could barely hide my despair regarding the tumor's aggressive activity described by the pathologist. Linden's big, blue eyes filled with tears as we spoke. It was hard to hold back my own tears. (I've always been a closet "wussy.") Jimmy just looked embarrassed. I knew he didn't understand the significance of positive tumor margins, stage C versus stage A, and so forth. He was also blessed with the natural immortality of youth.

The next few daylight hours at home were uneventful, but as twilight turned into dusk and the long shadows outside turned into darkness, I almost lost it again, emotions-wise. As I sat in my recliner watching TV, I suddenly noticed that the thick dressing on my low back was wet—the skin exit site from the epidural catheter. The catheter had been removed yesterday. I went into my bathroom and removed the dressing to examine it. The gauze was saturated with fluid—clear, odorless, colorless. Undoubtedly, leaking from subcutaneous infiltration from the previous infusion, I reasoned logically to myself. I carefully reapplied a fresh, sterile, dry dressing with some pressure. Thirty minutes later the new dressing was thoroughly and completely soaked. Objectively, I knew I was fine: no pain or discomfort, afebrile, completely asymptomatic; but I literally began to panic. My mind went through the list of really far out possibilities. I considered a spinal fluid leak leading to meningitis, possible midbrain herniation with developing paralysis, irreversible coma leading to inevitable death, and other even less likely horrors.

My mind began to race. I'm sure my pulse quickened. My hands began to perspire. I thought, I must get to the emergency room immediately! At the very least I need immediate rehospitalization for observation. I was certain the anesthesiologist on call would immediately inject a blood patch to stop the spinal fluid leak. This is a procedure in which a small amount of blood is withdrawn from a vein and injected into the deep tissue around the spinal puncture site. As the blood clots adjacent to the spinal fluid leak site, it "patches" the hole in the dura mater (the "durable" tissue that surrounds the spinal cord and contains the spinal fluid).

Now, my imagination was running wild. Naturally, I reasoned, I would require the infusion of massive antibiotics and intensive care unit (ICU) observation to survive—or to treat all my inevitable complications. I began to make mental preparations to rush to the hospital emergency room. Maybe an anesthesiologist who knows me will be available and not be busy doing a case in the O.R.

Then, with considerable effort, I objectively pictured myself in the presence of the E.R. physician who would evaluate me when I arrived with all my paraphernalia in tow. I visualized his reaction to my silly panic—and me a surgeon, at that. It was a struggle, but I managed to pull myself together and finally regain my aplomb. But the episode made me painfully aware that my nerves were frayed, big time.

Finally, as bedtime approached, I started to go through a set of rituals I would have to do nightly for the next two weeks. I would hate them progressively worse each night. First, I would clean around the Foley catheter with soap and water at its exit from my tender penis meatus. This removed mucous and debris (and subsequently pus) that had accumulated since the last time I cleaned it— generally three or four hours before. Next, I would don a clean pair of loose-fitting workout shorts (briefs, and even boxer shorts, were out of the question for the duration). Then, I would empty the urine from my leg bag, disconnect the bag from the catheter, and hook up the larger, less mobile, collection unit. This one could be suspended from my bed by hook, or simply laid on the floor next to the bed. It was large enough to collect urine overnight without danger of overflowing. Lastly, I would get into bed on my left side and carefully adjust the covers to allow some movement of the catheter tube. My objective was to accommodate myself in bed to eliminate excessive movement of the catheter or tubing. Although Dr. Williams had ingeniously secured the Foley catheter to my upper thigh to minimize trauma, it was impossible to achieve a completely immobile system.

Amazingly, I was usually able to fall asleep easily, and mostly slept through the night. However, the process became more onerous and uncomfortable as the days passed and the inevitable urethritis and meatitis developed (inflammation of the urethra secondary to the trauma of the catheter). The urethra was not meant to hold a solid foreign body (rubber tubing) irritating its fragile mucosa. Nature intended the urethra only for the intermittent, gentle passage of warm, physiologically neutral fluid over that tender and vulnerable tissue tube.

The Foley catheter was most bothersome during the day while I was most active. No movement or activity was possible without a payment of discomfort. Early on, the discomfort was mostly mild irritation. During the last days the catheter was in place, the result of accidental direct trauma or sudden traction was a spasm of teeth-clinching, severe pain. When Dr. Williams told me preoperatively that the worst thing about the radical prostatectomy operation was wearing a Foley catheter for three weeks, I could barely appreciate the truth of his message. But his assessment was right on. Every other inconvenience was no contest. Some urologists remove the catheter postoperatively as early as ten days to two weeks. Dr. Williams believed that his conservative approach decreased the necessity of having to reintroduce the catheter due to incomplete healing. He felt that the discomfort of wearing the catheter an extra week was justified to lessen the possible complications from removing the catheter too early. Due to my experience with my urethral stricture that subsequently developed, presumably secondary to catheter trauma, I question that "conservative" decision.

CHAPTER 14

He who has health, has hope; and he who has hope, has everything.

—Arabian Proverb

A theological pundit once remarked that so many coincidences happen because God wants to remain anonymous. A perfect example of this tenet occurred on my first morning at home after my surgery, Saturday, March 21. It's important to understand my mental state on that day. I was still emotionally stunned after reading my unexpectedly depressing pathology report the day before. And I've already alluded to the fact that surgeons make poor surgical patients because of their knowledge of all the operative complications and other bad things that are possible. Also, most doctors are prone to be fatalistic by nature. Whereas most patients have little concept of the difference in prognosis between a very favorable cancer and a very deadly cancer, most physicians are acutely aware of what is likely to be curable and what isn't. So I'm sure most members of my profession tend to view their own infirmities from the darker side. We've usually seen, or at least remember, too many patients or associates who did poorly.

On that Saturday morning I arose from bed and began to do what eventually became a routine. After combing my hair and shaving—the usual stuff—and arranging my tubes and paraphernalia for daytime activities, I made myself a large cup of flavored, sweet coffee and cream (General Foods's Cafe Vienna). Then, I settled myself in my La-Z-Boy recliner to leisurely drink the coffee and read the morning paper. This was the only time during the day I was likely to be comfortable and at peace with my environment. This morning interlude was such a pleasure during those troubled days that even now I still enjoy the ceremony of starting my day alone in the morning with coffee and the newspaper in my living room recliner.

On this Saturday morning I had switched the television on. A network talk show was in progress to which I was paying virtually no attention as I read the paper, enjoyed my coffee and tried to forget how sorry I felt for myself. The next guests introduced by the talk show host caused me to perk up my attention. They were Dr. Bernie Siegel, a surgeon, and one of his cancer patients. Dr. Siegel had written two popular books on the therapeutic value of cancer patients' developing the proper intellectual and emotional perspectives toward their disease. The patient represented an organization founded by the doctor called Exceptional Cancer Patients, or ECaP. She was a lady who had previously developed advanced breast cancer that had been cured. Although she had undergone traditional treatment for her malignancy, she believed that her treatment success was enhanced by the nontraditional supplemental methods advocated by Dr. Siegel. I listened intently as the former general surgeon expounded his controversial theory that natural immune mechanisms for controlling cancer and other diseases could be augmented by neuropeptides (enzymes) produced by the brain as a response to certain positive activities, thoughts, and routines. Although I had never previously considered such theories as legitimate therapy, my mental state then was such that I would consider anything short of snake oil and asafetida bags.

During the interview Dr. Siegel also alluded to a book written by Carl and Stephanie Simonton, of Texas. Their book, *Getting Well Again,* advocated theories similar to Siegel's. Unbeknownst to me then, some close friends were mailing me a copy of *Getting Well Again.* So I had coincidentally chanced upon a philosophy and program that I had previously never heard of, at a time when I was sorely in need of any type of positive support.

By the conclusion of the TV show I was intrigued with the positive message of hope expressed by Dr. Siegel and ECaP. I looked forward to examining his theories in greater detail. Later that same day I had Linden purchase Siegel's second book, *Peace, Love & Healing,* at my neighborhood WaldenBooks store. She placed a special order for his original book, *Love, Medicine & Miracles,* which was not in stock. Siegel's and the Simontons' writings would ultimately help me enormously in my recovery from surgery and, subsequently, radiation therapy. More important, they would change my whole outlook toward my future despite whether their teachings affected my ultimate recovery. The attitudes I developed while studying the lifestyles of the special people these authors described allowed me to enjoy life more than I would have ever hoped or imagined. Eventually, after considerable thought and study, I embraced their philosophy that made my physical and spiritual well-being "weller than well," to quote Dr. Siegel. I may die tomorrow or next century, but until I do, I'll remain Alive and Well!

CHAPTER 15

Often it is just a lack of imagination that keeps a man from suffering very much.

—Marcel Proust

My first full weekend at home following my operation was otherwise uneventful. After my Saturday evening panic attack I resolved to stay as mentally disciplined as possible. I developed patterns and routines to follow—some new ones and some from the past—that seemed to make me comfortable within the confinement of my situation. Like sitting in my recliner reading the newspaper and enjoying my first morning cup of coffee, for example. Another ritual I developed into an art: the morning transition from my nighttime catheter bag to my daytime leg bag, the opposite at bedtime.

Dr. Williams had scheduled an office appointment for me Monday, March 23, to remove my incision skin clips and, I hoped and dreaded, my remaining Jackson-Pratt drain. The drain output decreased to less than 40 cc daily over the weekend, so I was certain he would remove it. Remembering the transiently sickening discomfort when he had removed the first drain, I hoped I wouldn't embarrass myself with a display of nerves or other reflex reaction. Sure enough, he removed it. Sure enough, it was as unpleasant as I remembered. And sure enough, I remained poker-faced and motionless. Dr. Williams subtly acknowledged my stoicism as his eyes met mine immediately after the *coup de grâce*. He shook his head from side to side ever so slightly in admiration of my machismo. Only I knew the extent of my feigned bravery.

My incision was healing very well. Naturally, I expected the skin edges to fall apart when Dr. Williams removed the skin clips. They didn't. I knew I would surely develop an incision abscess that would lead to a full-blown incision hernia. Thankfully, I realized I would not likely have an evisceration since the operation was retroperitoneal and did not enter the peritoneal cavity. The peritoneal cavity houses the organs that eviscerate when this catastrophic incision failure happens. But I would undoubtedly develop a huge incision abscess that would extend deep into my pelvis, contain huge collections of foul-smelling pus, and require a major operation under anesthesia to properly drain it. I would assuredly need intravenous antibiotics to reduce the sepsis that would develop due to staphylococcus aureus ("staph") or other toxic bacteria. My active imagination conjured up the full spectrum of postoperative complications, but there was no evidence of any incision abnormality to my critical examination on that seventh postoperative day. It began to seem unlikely that I was going to develop any wound problem. I didn't. The incision healed rapidly and solidly, without even the slightest blemish.

Later, at home, it felt great to have an almost bare anterior abdominal surface. The only remaining semblance to naked skin and healthy scar on my pudgy, pale belly was a double strand of blue surgical suture. This suture was incongruently protruding through the skin just above my left groin. It was difficult to keep those six-inch-length segments bundled together beneath a gauze pad. They seemed to snake their way out no matter how securely I applied tape over the gauze. Their purpose was to allow safe introduction of another Foley catheter in case the first one fell out. The suture attached to the end of the catheter inside the bladder. It was brought to the skin surface through the bladder wall by a small stab incision. If the indwelling catheter balloon broke and the catheter fell out, a new catheter could be attached to the end of the suture exiting the penis. Then, the catheter could be pulled retrograde back through the urethra into proper position within the bladder. That technique would be much safer than probing the urethra blindly, thereby chancing an injury to the urethra-bladder anastomosis. It was an ingenious setup, but I'm happy that that insurance policy never had to be cashed in.

Being an active and dedicated runner (jogger) I was in excellent physical condition before my surgery except for marginally high body-fat percentage. A year earlier I had lost over twenty pounds and had conscientiously kept the weight off. I know that my good physical condition contributed greatly to my uneventful postoperative course, and it probably made my convalescence more comfortable. Since I was truly addicted to exercise, I now began to crave some physical activity. Against Linden's advice, I went for a half-mile walk in my neighborhood on a pleasant and warm Tuesday, March 24, my eighth postoperative day. It was exhilarating, and I did fine. I could have gone even further, but the irritation of my catheter made that consideration distinctly impractical. Nevertheless, I was pleased I could do that; and I was proud of myself.

For the next several days I continued to walk every day. I even pulled weeds in the yard once, which proved to be good stretching exercise and nonirritating to my sensitive private parts. By now I had begun to read Siegel's book. His writings had caused me to consider the possibility that I might not waste away and die a painful, cancer-ridden death within the next few weeks. I was still quite concerned, however, about the possibility—really the fact—that malignant cells were left behind in the prostate bed. How to deal with that reality was a question I was struggling with. But my subconscious was active during that period and would eventually sort things out for me.

On my first-week anniversary from hospitalization, my tenth postoperative day, I planned to visit my office briefly. Later, I learned that this was out of concert with Dr. Siegel's teachings, but it successfully directed my focus away from feeling sorry for myself. As medical director for the Texas Rehabilitation Commission, I had no private patients to whom I was directly responsible. That is, my current medical practice was administrative only. Before my surgery, my staff and I had been working several important rehabilitation policy initiatives that had been put on hold pending my recovery from surgery. Although none were critically time sensitive, I had committed to the commissioner that my office would produce these program policies by April 1. My staff had worked hard on these and was awaiting only my final approval. I was determined to try to meet that deadline, if possible.

Friday, March 27, I was the first customer in Roy's Village Flat Top Shop, a 1950's era barber shop throwback a few streets down from my office. A fresh haircut was necessary to me to legitimize my reentry into the world of the living. Roy and I weren't well acquainted, but we were on the same economic values wavelength. His clientele were not into "styling," and I was not into twenty-dollar haircuts. He fashioned a conservative businessman's haircut for me while explaining his offsprings' various social ills. I sanctioned his artistry with appreciative sounds and expressed appropriate sympathy for his problems with his rotten kids. I paid him ten dollars for his work, including the tip. Then, I went on to my office to see what had to be done. I hoped the commissioner was traveling or otherwise disposed, and that my other colleagues were equally out of pocket. That would allow me to do what was necessary to make things happen properly and assure that we would meet all deadlines with quality products. That done, I could get home to my friendly comfort station/support system. Everything worked out great.

The next few days were uneventful and almost pleasant if I could have ignored that damned catheter. I went back to my office March 31 to review final drafts of the programs due April 1. They were almost perfect. After making a few necessary corrections, my secretary produced the final products, and I proudly forwarded them to the commissioner. Later, I realized that my work and my preoccupation with meeting my promised deadline had made me forget, at least momentarily, that I was undoubtedly consumed with body-wide cancer eating away at my innards, etc., etc., etc.

About this time I realized how ridiculous it was to continue wallowing in my morbid, fatalistic attitude. I decided I would rather live and work and be productive than feel sorry for myself and die. So I set out to learn the best way to effect that possibility.

CHAPTER 16

An education isn't how much you have committed to memory, or even how much you know. It's being able to differentiate between what you do know and what you don't.

—Anatole France

With my newly evolving positive attitude toward life, I looked forward optimistically to Wednesday, April 1. Except for the irritation from the Foley catheter, which was now becoming a really messy proposition, I was feeling stronger and less prone to quick fatigability. Also, I felt exhilarated that none of my feared postoperative complications were coming to pass.

My new goal was to educate myself comprehensively about all aspects of prostate cancer, and my condition in particular. A little learning may be a dangerous thing, but an education is a shield of security. Today was the day I would start to build that shield.

After my morning rituals I drove myself to the Texas Medical Association Building at Fifteenth and Colorado streets in downtown Austin. I took the elevator to the medical library that encompasses most of the fifth floor. I had visited the library often in the past to review medical literature, usually relating to rehabilitation subjects. Today, my project was to get super-knowledgeable about prostate cancer. Specifically, I planned to learn everything about prostate cancer treated by radical prostatectomy for clinical stage A disease that turns out to be pathological stage C. I intended to learn about incidence, prognosis, and indications for adjunctive therapy; i.e. radiation and/

or chemotherapy. Also, I wanted to comprehend the significance of Gleason scoring, especially Gleason score 6–7—my score! Earlier at home, I had done a computer search of medical articles using PaperChase, a medical literature search service accessed through CompuServe. Using this technique, I had amassed the bibliographies of many promising articles to review. As a very enthusiastic computer buff, I had used CompuServe often in the past to access PaperChase. I was always impressed with the quality of their medical literature database.

After spending most of the morning in the TMA Library reviewing and learning, I partially accomplished my goal. I now knew a great deal about my disease and its variations. Most important, I learned that there was no pat answer to what next would be best for me. I had made a good start, but there was much more to learn. The easy accessibility to a men's rest room from the library allowed me to empty my leg bag as necessary, but it was an uncomfortable, very tiring morning. I had intended to spend more hours in study than I did, but it was obvious that my stamina was not up to the schedule my mind had programmed.

Experiencing the mental and emotional exhaustion that I had developed studying my personal, life-threatening disease and its implications for death and disability, I really felt like I needed some exercise. I decided to take my sand wedge to my golf course and see if I could relax by hitting a few easy practice balls on the golf practice range. I did that without apparent catastrophe, and it was quite relaxing, physically and mentally. My shots were amazingly straight and solid, confirming the golf experts' advice that you should swing easy for control and accuracy. I wasn't cavalier enough to try any longer clubs, and, in truth, I was tiring fast after twenty or twenty-five shots. But again, I felt Alive and Well!

Monday, April 6, my twenty-first postoperative day, Linden drove me to Dr. Williams' office for my scheduled appointment. The big day had come to remove my urinary catheter. Several times, and again on that day, Dr. Williams explained to me that the normal male urinary anatomy provided two sphincters that relaxed and contracted to control the urinary stream. The sphincter at the bladder neck was mostly involuntary. The other sphincter, located within the proximal urethra, was mostly a voluntary one. The bladder neck sphincter was normally "closed" until willed open by a man's conscious intention to urinate. The urethral sphincter tended to open passively when urged by urine pressure, but could shut off urine flow by one's positive intention. My anastomosis between the urethra and the bladder neck was upstream from my urethral sphincter, which had not been involved in my surgery. Although the operation effectively destroyed all semblances of the bladder neck sphincter, I should retain the ability to start and stop my urinary flow by conscious will. But since my urethral sphincter was my only control mechanism now, I would probably leak some urine with coughing or straining. Also, I may have variable urinary incontinence for a period. It may be very slight, but enough to require wearing absorbent pads. Apparently, the degree of incontinence and its duration varies considerably from patient to patient, and is most difficult to predict.

Before physically removing the catheter, Dr. Williams injected contrast media into the bladder through the catheter. Then, he released the fluid from the balloon part of the catheter within the bladder and asked me to strain as if voiding. I couldn't tell if I was successfully urinating around the catheter or not, which was the idea intended. The X-ray taken while voiding, however, showed the anastomosis to be intact and without leakage. The catheter slipped out easily and pain-free (surprise!). Next, Dr. Williams had me stand up to urinate (my stream could knock over a Coke bottle—just like when I was eighteen). Finally, he asked me to show how I could consciously stop the flow (I could, easily). No sweat! I felt great! I assured the good doctor I would probably be one of the few who had no problems at all with leakage or incontinence.

Despite my bravado with Dr. Williams about my incontinence potential, I really wasn't sure how great a problem I would have. It turned out I did do quite well. I never experienced any stress incontinence (losing urine with coughing or straining). I would frequently leak a small amount of urine, however, when I felt the urge to urinate and didn't promptly take measures to empty my bladder. This phenomenon, called urge incontinence, is less onerous than stress incontinence. Consequently, whenever I began to feel the urge to go, I went, and quickly. Although the volume voided each time was not great, I paid little attention to that at first. The urge seemed to develop quickly, and it was very demanding. Further, I was punished with wet drawers if I failed to pay prompt homage to my urge. Later, I noted that my average urination quantity was significantly less than it was preoperatively. Again, that was just a rough "guesstimate," since I hadn't measured my normal urine volume in years, if ever.

The rest of that week I took advantage of my sick leave time and continued to recuperate at home. In truth, I could have easily spent some time in the office as far as my physical condition was concerned. Nonetheless, I wanted to get a better handle on my urination demands, if possible. I also wanted a few days to savor the joy of not having that damned catheter! I began my aerobic running program again that week and did very well.

Monday, April 13, I came back into my office planning to work no more than half a day for the next week or so. Before surgery, Dr. Williams had told me to plan on six weeks off the job. I had passed that information on to my supervisors, so they were surprised that I could come to work, even part time, beginning my fifth week of convalescence. It was really quite therapeutic for me to get back into the office. Half a day was about right, since that didn't cause me any significant fatigue or side effects. Although overnight and two- to three-day travel periods were a big part of my usual job activities, I had planned to forego all trips until I recovered completely. That particular provision was my bargaining chip with Linden to get her approval to go back to work early. Except being ten pounds lighter, which I viewed as a plus, I was unaffected by outward appearances at this stage, as far as I could tell.

CHAPTER 17

Family life is too intimate to be preserved by the spirit of justice. It can be sustained by a spirit of love which goes beyond justice.

—Reinhold Niebuhr

Easter Sunday, April 19, was a very happy day. By now I was fully convinced I was going to live through my surgery experience, at least. Review of all the medical literature I had researched had lifted my spirits to a large extent, and I was beginning to feel some better about my prognosis. Although it wasn't great, neither was it as grim as I first assumed. Of major concern was the fact that now, from a medical standpoint, no expert was sure what was the best course of therapy for my particular condition; i.e. local tumor extension, no metastatic disease, and positive resection margins. The only remaining avenue I needed to take to complete my fact-finding efforts was to review my pathology specimen with the pathologist. I had scheduled an appointment with him for the next day. I was also strongly considering the possibility of a personal consultation with a prostate guru at some prestigious academic teaching center. My research had found the Departments of Urology at Stanford University, Duke University, and The Mayo Clinic the most likely top nominees. My thinking wasn't firm on that idea, however. Ultimately, I decided to forego a decision until I judged how confident I felt with the local medical community's talent and experience.

Those thoughts had little to do with the pleasantness of this Easter Sunday, however. Linden and I had gone out for Sunday Brunch to the Z' Tejas Grill, an outstanding local restaurant with great ambience. We thoroughly enjoyed a wonderful meal there. Later that afternoon, each of our children called to talk especially to Dad. This was distinctly unusual. Although their mother expects them to call home on Easter, the call is always directed mostly to Mom. She is the social parent and the one most excited about catching up on all the happenings of our distant flock. I usually get a token thirty seconds or so at the end of the conversation when everyone has become concerned about the length and price of the call. This time was different. Linden would answer the phone, shriek with delight, take and make perfunctory greetings, then look over at me, hand me the phone, and say, "It's for you. It's Valerie (Frank, Jim)!" And I would get all sorts of loving messages, expressions of concern and encouragement, and love. It was very nice. In the evening, as my wife and I were discussing the day and its moments, Linden looked at me and said, "You know, Honey, your kids sure love their daddy."

CHAPTER 18

Education is a progressive discovering of our ignorance.

—Will Durant

Monday, April 20, I drove to Seton Northwest Hospital to review my specimen pathology with Dr. Stewart, the pathologist assigned to my case. When I called him earlier to ask for a meeting to review my slides and discuss his findings, he was very gracious and willing to honor my request.

When I arrived at the hospital pathology department, Dr. Stewart had already marked pertinent areas on my tissue specimen slides for us to examine. Also, he had set up a teaching microscope for our dual use. This was a microscope with a special auxiliary set of eyepieces. That allowed the operator to control the movement and position of the slide while viewing the tissue. A second viewer could also examine the tissue through the other set of eyepieces at the same time.

When I examined my stained tumor tissue fixed on the prepared slides, I was instantly impressed by the bizarre architecture of the malignant cells. I was also impressed by their infiltration throughout the specimen. It was difficult (for me) to find a field of normal prostate histology to look at for comparison with the tumor cells. Also, I could see that the tumor was very, very close to the edge of the surgical resection in several areas. Of much greater concern, however, were the single and occasionally double cancer cells present outside the tumor mass within nerve bundles. This was usually indicative that the tumor was invading the perineural blood vessels and beginning to enter the blood stream. Had my lymphocytes—which I later came to image as my "mad-dog white cells"—done their job in destroying and devouring these cancer cells within the blood stream? Or could some have survived and taken up residency in other organs and tissues? Only time would tell, but the prospects were chilling.

Dr. Stewart was exceptionally kind and cordial to me during our brief introductory exchange, but he was candid in his description of his findings in my specimen. I knew that his examination of my tumor made him dubious about my chances for a clear-cut cure from surgery alone. As we examined various areas of my specimen and the tumor's characteristics, we discussed the possible value of other treatment, such as adjuvant radiation or chemotherapy. Although he admitted he was not a clinician, Dr. Stewart confirmed that if he were in my situation, he would not procrastinate in seeking further treatment, if available and feasible.

My next appointment with Dr. Williams was for the next day, Tuesday, April 21. Based on my meeting with Dr. Stewart, I planned to ask him to recommend to me another prostate cancer specialist with whom I could discuss my case. I envisioned an expert who was an established authority in all phases of prostate cancer management and, in addition, someone who didn't know me from Adam. This latter criterion would allow, I hoped, an unemotional, abstract evaluation of my present condition. More important, this superspecialist would recommend what further treatment, if any, was appropriate, now or in the future, for my particular situation, age, general health status, etc. Subsequently, Dr. Williams offered the names of several giants in the field of urology. He agreed to refer me to one or more. Presumably, the chosen consultant and I would discuss whether or not more than just a telephone consultation process was necessary. Alternatively, I would travel to their "Ivory Tower" office, probably carrying pathology slides and laboratory results in hand. I knew the latter would be very expensive. Considering the stakes involved, however, the prospect of my spending a few hundred dollars for that service was not a serious concern to me. Dr. Williams and I decided that we both needed more time to consider the specifics of this plan, considering the importance of whatever actions we take. At least there was no necessity to make a hasty decision.

Since I was now five weeks postoperative, Dr. Williams thought the time was right to get a follow-up serum prostate specific antigen (PSA) determination. His technician took a blood sample for that study before I left the office. Obviously, since I now had no prostate tissue at all, the test was expected to show no detectable antigen. Any value of PSA could only mean one thing—prostate cancer cells somewhere in the body producing antigen. I wasn't greatly concerned that the test would show any abnormality at this stage. My preoperative metastatic workup had been negative, so any free cancer cells floating around in the margins of my surgery area would not be of sufficient volume to produce a detectable antigen value yet. That is what I told myself intellectually. Emotionally, I didn't have a great deal of confidence in that logic. Very important, however, was my profound realization that this test was a sword of Damocles hanging interminably over my head. I would have to live with PSA tests from now until I die, or until a PSA finally comes back positive, confirmatory of cancer recurrence or metastasis. This awareness suddenly hit me like a flash of lightning. I am now sentenced for life to being periodically tested for a death commitment. I'm committed lifelong to the anxiety of having to sweat out the results of each test to know if my mortality is measured.

With all those happy thoughts in mind, I was grateful to Vernon M. Arrell, the commissioner of TRC, for inviting me to go on a spring turkey hunt with some mutual friends at a private ranch retreat. I wasn't physically able to actually hunt, nor did I really want to. But the quiet solitude of the lovely, isolated ranch and the relaxing environment of the Texas hill country were perfect for my heady deliberations about my future.

Earlier that week I had returned to full-time work at my agency. Although I had several important work issues to address, even those were therapeutic, I discovered. I walked around the ranch a lot that weekend with my rifle in tow, but I never fired a shot. Nonetheless, I was most invigorated when the trip was over. Paradoxically, the peacefulness of the isolated ranch lifted my spirits to the extent that I didn't feel quite so distanced from humankind just because I had "cancer."

The day after I got home from the hunting trip, I played golf with my regular group. Although I played poorly, I enjoyed their awe and astonishment that I could recover from major surgery so quickly. Later, Linden and I had our first deep and absorbing discussion regarding my prognosis. For most of our married life I had shared my innermost thoughts and concerns with my wife, who was also my best friend. On that evening we talked about my fear that there might still be malignant cells present in my pelvis, and what I was going to do about it. We also talked about my eternal slavery to laboratory tests and their results.

And we also talked about my impotence. Would that flaccid little organoid ever stand up again? Certainly not for several weeks/months/years (ever?). "That's the least of my concerns," she told me with conviction, and I know that is true; but it's a real concern to me, nevertheless—much more so than she could comprehend. Although Linden nor I had needed sex regularly for years, my psyche wanted the assurance that I could be a husband to my wife whenever the occasion came up, so to speak.

How does a man resign himself to losing something so emotionally charged as the ability to do sexual intercourse? Linden found this very difficult to understand; presumably because she's a woman, and sexual potency is a man thing. Jeff Nightbyrd, an excellent newspaper columnist for the *Austin* (Texas) *American-Statesman*, recently quoted a female critic: "Women are supposed to be unstable because they have a monthly cycle. But men are ruled by testosterone. Wherever their sex organs point, their mind follows." Jeff agrees: "Men discover themselves in infancy, and are still talking about sex on the way to the grave."

CHAPTER 19

Knowledge is knowing that we cannot know.
—Ralph Waldo Emerson

The following Tuesday I traveled to Dallas to attend a scheduled Physical Disabilities Workshop. This is a TRC-sponsored program given periodically for the education of vocational rehabilitation counselors and their administrative technicians. Various physical disabilities are discussed in relation to their etiology, prognosis, and potential for vocational rehabilitation. As a part of my job I attend these programs and serve as host and technical consultant for the medical professionals who give the formal presentations. After my initial welcoming address and orientation, my part of the program is largely unstructured. Within certain parameters I can come and go as I please.

For this workshop my priorities didn't allow me to attend many conference sessions. As I had intended, I spent most of each day in the huge medical library of the University of Texas Southwestern Medical School. My education about prostate cancer now centered on my becoming a knowledgeable authority on adjunctive therapy. I was especially interested in adjuvant therapy for pathologic stage C adenocarcinoma of the prostate initially treated surgically—my prostate cancer.

The most recent medical literature confirmed what I had learned previously: Approximately forty percent of clinical stage A prostate cancer turns out to be pathologic stage C. Next, I learned that there was no consensus of the top medical authorities in any clinical specialty regarding what adjunctive therapy, if any, was useful for that (my) situation. I already knew that either radical surgery or ablative radiation therapy gave equally good results for clinical stage A prostatic carcinoma for ten years after treatment, according to most studies. After ten years the radiation-treated groups developed higher recurrence rates than the surgery-treated patients. Consequently, primary radiation was usually recommended for older patients and patients with higher surgical risk factors. Radical prostatectomy was generally recommended for younger men. In patients who had distant metastases already, hormones were the palliative (symptomatic) treatment of choice. Curative treatment was not a rational goal in the situation where a tumor had already spread to distant organs, such as bones, liver, or lungs.

For several good reasons, medical experts were unsure what to do next, if anything, after radical prostatectomy for a pathologically proven stage C prostate cancer. Firstly, the radical prostatectomy operation itself had evolved dramatically in the last several years due to better understanding of the surgical anatomy, improved operative techniques, and better anesthesia. Because of these factors, today's surgical patients cannot be compared qualitatively to the surgical patients of a few years ago. Next, adjunctive radiation therapy using the powerful new linear accelerators provides radiation doses that are much higher and more accurately directed than were possible several years ago. The new machines are also associated with fewer complicating side effects than the cobalt units of a decade ago. Because of these radical changes in the quality of treatment available today, it will take several more years to learn whether adjuvant radiation will improve survival in stage C prostate cancer patients. These revelations made it apparent that there was no clear answer to my dilemma: Should I opt for further treatment; that is, adjuvant radiation?

That evening I had dinner with an old friend, my former organic chemistry professor in undergraduate school at Southern Methodist University. Dr. Harold Jeskey had also been my premedical course advisor, and he was instrumental in my being accepted to several prestigious medical schools. I intended to tell him about my prostate cancer, accept his sympathy and condolences, and generally wallow in my own self-pity. Unfortunately for my ego, he didn't cooperate. Dr. Jeskey accepted my news with some alacrity, and then deftly shifted the subject. After that, we spent most of the evening discussing the recent loss of his wife of forty-plus years. I was disappointed about not getting my strokes, but I couldn't help being impressed with how my wily old professor had instigated our role reversal. Later, I could laugh at myself about my expectations for his sympathy and how I had been emotionally outmaneuvered by a pro.

Friday, I returned to my office from Dallas. Dr. Williams had not called and left me any message. Forthwith, I called his clinical laboratory directly and asked for the result of my PSA test. The antigen was undetectable.

The following Wednesday I visited with Dr. Williams in his office. After some mutual discussion, we both agreed that I should have adjunctive radiation therapy. Again, we knew there was no hard or soft scientific evidence that showed this regimen would increase my chance for a cure. It just seemed logical to both of us that since my pathology examination strongly suggested that microscopic tumor had been left behind, my prostate bed needed to be zapped. We hoped the radiation would destroy any remaining malignant cells before they had a chance to grow or spread. Several major research centers were currently doing prospective, double-blind studies to see if local radiation would improve the cure rate. I had no desire to be a part of such a study. I didn't want to chance being blindly selected for the "control" group and not have the option to control my treatment choice. Nor did I feel inclined to wait patiently for twenty years until the research studies had resolved the issue.

I learned from my readings in Dallas that although supplemental radiation had not improved cure rates in the past (from studies using the older X-ray units), that treatment significantly decreased cancer recurrences in the pelvis. Although I had no evidence to suggest it, I couldn't be completely sure I didn't already have microscopic seeding of tumor cells to my bones or other internal organs. If so, these microscopic metastases would inevitably progress to gross metastatic disease eventually.

But if I were destined to have recurrent cancer, I assuredly didn't want it to show up in my pelvis. Recurrent malignancy in this anatomic area could cause possible bowel or bladder obstruction requiring a colostomy or urinary diversion procedures for "palliation." These complications are the most unpleasant, abhorrent consequences of treatment failure. I was quite willing to face the risks and problems associated with radiation therapy to avoid the possibility of cancer recurrence in the pelvis.

Dr. Williams gave much forethought to which of several local radiation therapy doctors he would recommend to me. He felt that I should choose a radiation oncologist with whom I would be completely compatible. This was because I would be under that doctor's direct care daily for at least six weeks during the radiation treatment. Undoubtedly, I would experience some side effects, at least minor ones, that would need treatment, so I needed to trust and respect my new doctor's judgment. Dr. Williams named two radiation oncologists with whom he had developed a positive professional relationship and recommended them for my consideration. I interviewed both.

The first physician was an older doctor (my age). During my initial appointment he took my medical history and did a physical examination. I thought the physical examination was perfunctory and less than useful. Although he found no anorectal abnormality on examination (and I gave no history of colon problems), he said he wanted me to have a barium enema or colonoscopy (my choice) before beginning the anticipated radiation therapy. I assumed that was standard procedure, so I called a local gastroenterologist and arranged for a colonoscopy.

The second radiation therapist I visited, Dr. John H. Wilbanks, was frank, candid, positive—a real "can-do" person—and up-to-date clinically and academically, by my evaluation. I chose him. He saw no indication for a colon evaluation, so I canceled the colonoscopy. My bowel wasn't a concern to me. First things first. One problem at a time. Let's get on with the treatment. Charge!

CHAPTER 20

Science is simply common sense at its best—that is, rigidly accurate in observation, and merciless to fallacy in logic.

—Thomas Huxley

My first radiation treatment appointment was scheduled for Monday, May 18, at the Shivers Radiation Treatment Center in Austin, almost exactly two months after my prostate surgery. The center was the namesake of former Texas governor Allan Shivers, himself a cancer victim. Dr. Wilbanks, my new radiation oncologist, had encouraged me to bring Linden to my first session and to be prepared to ask questions.

The first order of business at the center, naturally, was my filling out insurance forms and other necessary paperwork. Then, I was escorted to the treatment simulator room while Linden waited in the outer waiting room. After donning a standard hospital smock, I was asked to lie down on the table of the treatment simulator. This apparatus was a very sophisticated mock treatment machine used to carefully define the treatment target area for radiation therapy using body positioning, X-ray views, and other measurement techniques. This initial session consisted of approximately two hours of painstaking fittings and measurements, carefully orchestrated by Dr. Wilbanks and the center's professional staff assigned to this extremely important function. Finally, after my positioning was perfect, Dr. Wilbanks directed the placement of three small tattoo markers. These dots were indelibly marked on my hips bilaterally at precisely determined landmark bisections and at my pubis in the midline, anteriorly. During my actual treatments these marks would be used to meticulously align me to the radiation unit using laser light beam guides for precision positioning.

Before beginning my regimen of therapy, the center radiation physicist would analyze all the sophisticated data that were measured using the simulator. Based on that analysis, the radiation treatment dose to my prostate bed would be calculated. He would also calculate the radiation dose to the margin areas—those peripheral points just outside the prostate bed, including the surrounding pelvic structures.

Dr. Wilbanks explained that my treatment plan would consist of 6,120 rads (units of radiation) directed to the prostatic bed in my pelvis. He could precisely target that point because Dr. Williams had marked the area at surgery using metallic clips visible on X-rays. With modern treatment techniques and a very powerful linear accelerator (the most powerful radiation unit available in Austin), 95 percent of the radiation dose would be confined to a two-centimeter margin of the pelvis where the prostate previously resided anatomically. This would be done by rotating the radiation treatment arm over a 270 degree span, sparing the most anterior 45 degrees and the posterior 45 degrees of my pelvis. That technical maneuver would effectively minimize radiation to the bladder (anterior) and rectum (posterior). Because of the linear accelerator technology, radiation to overlying skin would be negligible. This advantage of minimal skin irradiation was in contrast to the older cobalt-60 radiation unit. With the cobalt machine, the dose delivered to the desired area was limited to the amount of radiation the skin could tolerate. The cobalt unit still has considerable usefulness for treatment of many head and neck cancers and breast cancers, but is outmoded for effective treatment of most deep-seated tumors.

Linden and I had compiled many questions to ask our new doctor-therapist if he gave us the opportunity. After all the treatment simulator measurements were complete, she and I settled down in the doctor's office to give him the third degree. Thankfully, Dr. Wilbanks was very patient and helpful. He thoughtfully and willingly answered all our questions without hesitation or hint of patronization. Foremost in my mind was my concern about the relative quality of the radiation treatment technology in Austin compared with a university center— in Houston, Dallas, or elsewhere. Dr. Wilbanks readily convinced me that the available technology in Austin was outstanding, and at least equal to any major medical center anywhere in the Southwest or elsewhere.

Earlier, I had probed Dr. Wilbanks about my proposed radiation dosage. In my medical research, one treatment center in California recommended 4,000 rads for patients in similar circumstances. Dr. Wilbanks expressed the strong conviction (as did the "medical world," he said) that the appropriate dose was near 6,000 rad. "Then why not exactly 6,000 rads," I asked, "instead of 6,120?"

"Simple rounding off," he replied. "We want to deliver a minimum of 6,000 rads. Each daily treatment will deliver 180 rads tumor dose. We'll try to give five treatments per week to a total of thirty-four. Total dose would be 180 rads times thirty-four treatments equals 6,120 rads. One fewer treatments would not deliver the 6,000 rads minimum required dose."

"Why specifically five treatments per week? And what happens if something causes me to miss a treatment?" were my next questions.

"Experts in some parts of the country go on a four-day-per-week treatment cycle," Dr. Wilbanks explained, "and that may be okay. We really don't know for sure. But radiation physics theory and cell biology predict that the best tumorcidal dose of radiation and the best recovery patterns for normal cells favor five doses per week. We don't get too upset if somebody misses one or two days in a six-week treatment regimen, but we get a little nervous if treatment drags out long enough to average closer to four treatments per week than five."

Next, I wondered, "Even with those indelible tattoos on my skin and the compulsive positioning to line up the marks properly before each treatment, how do you know for sure that the treatment is being delivered to the same place each time?"

He quickly replied, "We'll shoot a pelvic X-ray to verify proper positioning at least once weekly, sometimes more often, just to make sure we're still consistent in the radiation treatment target. But we seldom have to adjust because of the skill and competence of our radiation technicians."

Dr. Wilbanks then carefully explained to us the normal effects and potential side effects to be anticipated because of treatment. He discussed the fact that all radiation therapy will produce mild general symptoms, also several specific symptoms common to radiation of certain anatomic locations. And the side effects are quite variable from individual to individual. Some patients never complain or admit to any side effects, but some transient problems should always be anticipated. Weight loss during treatment is common, for example, so he recommended a nutritious, high-protein, low-fat diet and multivitamin supplements. "This isn't the time to go on a rigid, weight-reduction diet," Dr. Wilbanks emphasized.

Anemia and leukopenia (low white blood cells) sometime occur during radiation therapy, but are much more likely to develop in patients who get treatment to wider areas of the body and encompassing considerable bone marrow—for example, the spine and pelvis. "We'll get routine weekly blood counts during treatment, but I seriously doubt if you'll have any problems in this regard since the treatment is closely focused to your prostate bed." Dr. Wilbanks continued, "I expect your most likely side effects will be related to the bladder and rectum. In this treatment there's no way we can avoid irradiating the anterior wall of the rectum and the perianal area. Also, a variable amount of bladder wall will get irradiated." He told us I could expect some perianal itching to begin toward the end of the second week of treatment. The symptoms may later simulate an exacerbation of acute hemorrhoids. I told him I had never had any trouble with hemorrhoids. He just smirked.

"You might also expect to develop increased urinary frequency and urgency," he continued. I couldn't imagine how I could develop any more frequency and urgency than I already had. My urgency to urinate was so marked that I had learned to stake out all the available restrooms any time I went anywhere. And any attempt to try to postpone urination after the first urge invariably turned out to be a serious mistake. This, and my diminishing urinary stream caliber, were not normal postoperative expectations, but I didn't realize it then.

I had my initial treatment three days later, Thursday, May 21. While setting up for the procedure, I wondered aloud to a radiation technician why my treatment had not begun the day after my simulation visit three days earlier. "You had your simulation just Monday?" he exclaimed with surprise. "You must have gotten a real rush job on the physics. It usually takes at least a week for the radiation physicist to make all the calculations before treatment." Rank has its privileges, I suppose.

CHAPTER 21

Where there is the necessary technical skill to move mountains, there is no need for the faith that moves mountains.

—Eric Hoffer

The Shivers Radiation Treatment Center in East Austin is located in a largely African-American neighborhood consisting mostly of older single-family homes and an occasional small neighborhood business. The area is not a ghetto, but it is definitely not a ritzy section of town. The center is housed in an unimposing medium-sized, single-story, stone building. The simple landscaping and central parking lot are always clean and well maintained, in contrast to many adjacent buildings and homes. Upon entering the building from the front parking lot, the reception desk where patients sign in is on the right, just inside the door. Regular "customers" are always warmly greeted by name by the receptionist, a very kind and polite matronly lady.

Every patient is assigned a designated treatment time. Mine was 2:00 P.M. daily. On my first treatment day I arrived at 1:45, signed the register and sat down in the waiting room. I was new and unrecognized, but the receptionist treated me with utmost politeness and respect. Later, I would become a known regular and get the warmer reception by name. The waiting room was not small, but was barely adequate for the patient volume. The furniture was a mix and match, but the chairs were all comfortable. An inviting pot of coffee and plastic cups were available in the central area. There were also several children-sized chairs and tables and an adjacent large wooden box stuffed with remnants of difficult-to-damage toys. These served as somber reminders that cancer was heartless in its choice of victims. I was struck by a huge painting titled *The Pool at Bethesda* that occupied one entire wall. An adjacent plaque explained the legend of the pool: An angel from heaven appeared periodically at the pool and granted good health to ill or infirm petitioners who entered the waters. It was a very beautiful and relaxing painting that I would gaze at daily over the next several weeks and would get to know very well in every detail. It was months later that I learned that the pool at Bethesda was of biblical origin:

> Now there is at Jerusalem by the sheep market a pool, which is called in the Hebrew tongue Bethesda, having five porches.
> In these lay a great multitude of impotent folk, of blind, halt, withered, waiting for the moving of the water.
> For an angel went down at a certain season into the pool, and troubled the water: whosoever then first after the troubling of the water stepped in was made whole of whatsoever disease he had. (John 5:2–4)

The pool at Bethesda was subsequently written into a short play in 1928 by Thornton Wilder, titled *The Angel That Troubled the Waters.*

At promptly 2:00 P.M. the receptionist called my name and instructed me to "go on back." I didn't yet know where "on back" was, so I was directed to the treatment area in the rear section of the building. A central nurse's station intersected the hallway from the waiting room and an adjacent hallway at right angles. The various treatment rooms lined this back hallway. I was directed to the last room on the right. As I approached the entryway to my treatment room I was greeted by two pleasant young men who introduced themselves as the radiation therapists assigned to my room. The younger one, Carl, would soon rotate to another area; but Neil was permanently assigned to my room for the duration of my therapy. I would learn that the junior radiation therapist/technician, Carl initially, rotated at intervals to different treatment rooms to gain experience with different types of tumors and their treatment regimens. The senior therapist, Neil, was permanently assigned to one treatment unit.

I was instructed to lie down on a treatment table—similar to a standard medical examination bed—that was a part of the large radiation treatment unit. It was more comfortable than the usual examination table because of a thin, overlying mattress. Next, I was asked to lower my trousers below my groin. As I did so, Carl was ready with a small towel to cover my genitalia, yet allowing exposure of my indelibly applied tattoo marks laterally and at my suprapubic midline. While I tried to settle into a comfortable position, I was instructed to move up several inches, now to the right, now slightly to the left. "Okay," said Neil, "now let us move you, and don't you try to help." By deftly manipulating a previously placed folded sheet beneath my bottom, they lifted my torso and fine-tuned my position until my tattoo marks exactly lined up with laser-light cross beams built into the machine. When Carl and Neil were satisfied with my position, they gave each other the thumbs up sign. Then, as if by signal, both strode resolutely out of the room without fanfare, leaving me completely alone. Before I had a chance to panic, Neil's voice resonated softly but clearly from a speaker on the room wall. "We're ready to go now, Dr. Payne. Lie perfectly still, but you can breathe normally. We can see you over our video monitor and can hear you if you have anything to say, so let us know if you have any problems. Otherwise, we'll come back in the room when your treatment is over."

As I laid there alone in the room, perfectly still as instructed, I looked at my surroundings as best I could from my supine position to fix the environment in my memory. The large treatment room walls and ceiling were painted off-white and were barren of fixtures or ornaments. The treatment machine was roughly in the center of the room. Earlier, it had impressed me by its imposing size and shape. It consisted of the patient table that was attached at the head to a large, gray, box-like structure with several huge bundles of electrical cables exiting. There was an elongated L-shaped appendage attached to a large circular base within the machine head. The base was marked with degree calibrations from 0 to 360. The limb of the "L" projected below my body level on the right side and extended several feet caudad (toward my feet). Apparently, it was designed to rotate across my body from lower right to lower left a preprogrammed number of degrees.

After lying there for what seemed like an eternity without anything happening (realistically, maybe two or three minutes) the machine began to emit a low-pitched whirring noise. A few seconds later the whirring changed to a distinct and continuing high-pitched crackle/buzz. Out of the corner of my right eye I could see that the L-arm of the machine had begun to slowly rotate up and over my right side. I was obviously being zapped, but I felt nothing, which was a semisurprise. Admittedly, I didn't know what to expect, but I thought I might feel some warmth, or maybe a tingling sensation. I felt nothing. The zapping, buzzing, moving arm continued to rise slowly upward around my body until it reached its preset limit of 45 degrees short of midline. Then, after a few seconds of silence, the arm let out a wheeze and moved again to set itself to the left of my midline, presumably 45 degrees again. After a few more seconds of inactivity and silence, the whirring started again, and was soon replaced by the crackle. The arm then began its descent to my left and downward until it was out of sight. A few seconds later: silence. Neil and Carl then waltzed back into the room. "That's it, Dr. Payne. We'll see you tomorrow; same time, same place."

The whole process had taken no longer than three minutes, less than two minutes of which was actual treatment time.

I sat up, climbed down from the table, and started to raise my pants to zip and button. First, though, I found myself curiously inspecting my genitalia and lower pelvis. I guess I expected to see smoke, or at least a red glow. Nothing was different or remarkable. That routine continued until the end of the week. Saturday and Sunday were treatment holidays.

I felt no side effects at all after the first six or seven sessions. It was about then that I had a scheduled consultation with the radiation-center dietitian, according to center policy. Her office was one of several in the administrative section of the center. It was small and unkempt. The walls held several charts displaying different properties of various food groups. A small bookcase contained typical, dietary-oriented texts. The dietitian told me, in essence, to avoid nuts and seeds and to maintain a low-residue diet. I viewed this advice with some skepticism since I didn't comprehend the rationale and had preached the sermon of high-fiber intake for years. Not until later in my course of treatment was I willing to accept her advice as worthwhile.

I had begun to do various little things during my treatments to occupy my mind. For instance, I used the stopwatch on my chronograph to check out the exact time of the radiation delivery (zapping treatment arm's rotation). Also, I had discovered that if I closed my left eye, I would see the treatment arm stop just short of a loose piece of ceiling tile I had become acquainted with. After the treatment arm moved across my front, it would stop near a label on a ceiling rail. It was comforting to me that these constants never varied during my entire course of treatment.

After every fifth or sixth session, Neil would ask me to remain in place on the table after my treatment to make an X-ray for a position check. Later, Dr. Wilbanks and I would have a short, weekly conference, and he usually commented that the X-rays showed proper positioning for perfect therapy. One technician always weighed me every Monday before my first treatment of the week. I also had a blood count done every Tuesday as a routine. My weight remained stable early on, and, as expected, my blood count was never affected by my therapy. Dr. Wilbanks explained again, "The radiation covers such a small amount of bone marrow, I'd be very surprised if you showed any bone marrow suppression." I actually gained a couple of pounds during the later stages of treatment.

I became well acquainted with my radiation therapists during my course of treatment, and I learned much technical information about my machine from Neil, most of which I didn't understand. For instance, my unit was called a Clinac 1800, manufactured by the Varian Company. It was a dual photon, dual modality type of treatment unit capable of delivering either 6 megavolts or 18 megavolts; or 6, 9, 12, 16, or 20 millivolt electrons. Trust me; this was quite powerful. I was receiving my treatment at, 18 megavolts, which allowed transmission of a well-directed deep, surface-sparing radiation dose. My understanding was that more superficial tumors would lend themselves to treatment using the six-megavolt delivery mode, much like the Cobalt-60 machine that was still being used at the Shivers Center in another room. Neil thought that some university centers used a machine called a Varian 2100 capable of delivering up to 2,100 megavolts, although he didn't know what its utility would be beyond the "1800." In addition, the Shivers Center had a Linac 4 linear accelerator of 4-megavolt capacity and a Sieman Mevatron, with 10-megavolt capacity. I never saw either of these in actual use.

My first radiation side effect developed insidiously Monday, June 1, after my seventh treatment. It consisted of only mild, but persistent, pruritus ani (anal itching). At first, I assumed I had been less than thorough with my postbowel-movement cleansing—I've done that, but when the itch continued unabated despite my best corrective treatment, I began to deduce the truth. But if an itching anus was to be my only side effect, I could handle that! The next day I had an episode of unexplained diarrhea. That made me very uneasy about what problems the future might hold, but except for one subsequent episode several weeks later, I had no more diarrhea per se. But the itching was quickly replaced by a very demanding inability to postpone defecation once I first experienced the urge. This inconvenience continued throughout the course of my radiation therapy and persisted for almost three weeks after my last treatment.

My radiation-induced bowel urgency caused only one notable "accident." This occurred early one morning at the office and was a distinctly uncouth experience, although it could have been much worse. I had arrived early at my office and was working at my desk trying to finish a short project when my colon sent my brain an emergency message that was the physiological equivalent of a warning shot across the bow. I made the distinct mistake of continuing to work for a little while longer. Before I could do much more than curse my poor judgment, I was incontinent of feces at my desk. Then, I was scrambling awkwardly down the hall to the nearest toilet, some fifty feet away. Fortunately, my secretary had not yet come in for the day. Mercifully, the hall was empty, so no one observed my considerable distress and duress as I hopscotched disjointedly into the john. It took a good while to control my chagrin, regain my composure and clean up the mess in my undershorts. Thankfully, the mess didn't leak through to my trousers before I could intervene. If it had, that would have been an intolerable situation to face. I had other close calls, but being highly coachable, I learned well from that one mistake. Otherwise, even that was a tolerable problem I could live with. But worse things were yet to come.

An interesting anecdote occurred after my fourth week of radiation. Linden and I and our older son, Frank, who was home on vacation, had dinner at a popular, highly rated Austin restaurant. Linden had clipped a discount ticket for the "Early Bird Special." My son and I had beef, but Linden had a broiled fish special that turned out to be a leftover from yesterday's menu. It was the second time we had eaten there, and we hadn't really enjoyed our meal the first time. Only because of the restaurant's outstanding reputation did we decide to give it a second try. Later that evening my wife became severely nauseated and vomited for several hours, almost surely due to the tainted fish. Frank and I had no such problem. The next morning Linden was fine, but she told me she had the most realistic dream. She said Dr. Bernie Siegel, the author of the books on cancer survival, had come to her in a dream. He told her she had chosen to become sick with nausea and vomiting "so Jim would not have to get sick due to the effects of his radiation treatment."

By four and one-half weeks into my therapy, I was becoming increasingly concerned regarding the frequency of my treatments. Earlier, Dr. Wilbanks had placed great emphasis on the necessity of a five-treatment-per-week regimen. For various reasons, after eighteen sessions from May 21 to June 19, I had never had more than four treatments per week. Then, during the week of June 22, my radiation machine broke down sometime after my Monday treatment and continued inoperative through Wednesday. When I expressed my concerns about treatment frequency to Dr. Wilbanks, he also became concerned, and resolved that I shouldn't miss any more treatment days under any circumstances. For that Thursday, he arranged for me to have my treatment at another radiation center in Austin using a somewhat less powerful machine. He assured me that it was no big deal to have one maverick treatment. The repairs were completed on my machine at the Shivers Center by the next day, so I had only one outside treatment. Of greater import to my fragile psyche, however, was that another treatment week had passed and this time I had had only three treatments. Since the next week would include the Independence Day holiday Friday, Dr. Wilbanks scheduled me to have five treatments in that four-day week.

After twenty-six of my scheduled thirty-four treatments, by July 3 I had developed a rip-roaring radiation proctitis that felt like the worst case of hemorrhoids you can imagine. I had also developed worsening symptoms of radiation cystitis, but the anorectal symptoms were so offensive, I scarcely noticed the urinary urgency, frequency, and my markedly weaker urinary stream. Because my perianal area had become exquisitely sore and tender, each bowel movement felt like salty razor blades seasoned with red pepper. It was precisely at this time that I recalled the dietitian's earlier admonition that I maintain a low-residue diet. I decided just then it might be worthwhile to heed her advice. Gratefully, this diet modification worked wonders, supplemented with hemorrhoidal ointment and hydrocortisone rectal suppositories. These medications had only been marginally effective before I began the low-residue diet. I still experienced significant anal discomfort and moderate bleeding with bowel movements, but the symptoms had become tolerable, due to my careful diet modification. These problems continued to a greater or lesser extent through the next two weeks, and my eight final treatments.

After my last treatment on July 15, I met with Dr. Wilbanks for a short outbriefing. He explained that the side effects of the treatment would begin to moderate over the next two weeks or so. They did, and by August 1 my anorectal symptoms were minimal. They didn't dissipate completely, however, until early September. Even by then my decreased bladder capacity and weak urine stream hadn't improved. Because I now had so many lesser things to complain about, I began to take greater notice of my continuing urinary problems. It was fortunate for me that I did.

CHAPTER 22

Pain adds rest unto pleasure, and teaches the luxury of health.

— Martin F. Tupper

August 1992 was a very enjoyable month for me and relatively uneventful from a medical standpoint. I was working full time at my job and had successfully completed several important work projects that had been placed on hold during my radiation treatment. I felt strong and healthy except for persistent arthritis symptoms in my right neck and shoulder, both hands, and both wrists. These aches and pains weren't new and weren't severe enough to limit my thrice-weekly running program nor my weekly golf game. My urinary symptoms were essentially unchanged: My urine stream was quite weak, and I had to go quickly when nature advised me I had to go. As with almost any disability, I suppose, I had become accustomed to the problem.

Several weeks previously, Linden and I had tentatively planned to drive to Gaylord, Michigan, during the third week of August. During this holiday we would visit friends and I would play in the National Left-Handed Golfers' Association National Championship Tournament. We did that and had a great time both coming and going, although I experienced a few problems. Several times during the road travel I came dangerously close to losing my urine control, or at least wetting my drawers. These episodes always occurred when I would make the mistake of not planning ahead accurately in my rest room rendezvous routine. I always made it, but occasionally I had to jump out of the car and bolt for the toilet leaving Linden to park or pump gas. She never complained.

It was impossible to predictably contemplate the

rapidity with which the urge to urinate would develop. It would progress from an almost indiscernible feeling of beginning bladder discomfort to a literally unbearable, raw-nerved, pressure pain within a precious few minutes. The pain would become so intense that I sometimes seriously considered whipping it out in broad daylight to get relief and take my chances later with the social consequences. Really!

My golf skill during the tournament left a lot to be desired, but my poor play was nothing unusual. Unfortunately, I couldn't blame my urinary tract for my poor golf scores.

After our return from Michigan, I scheduled a routine appointment with Dr. Williams for September 1. I reported that my urinary stream was gradually getting weaker and weaker and that I had recently begun to strain to assure that I had emptied my bladder completely. He knew that I had experienced the problem of urinary urgency since the day my catheter was removed after my operation. He also knew my symptoms worsened some during my course of radiation therapy. The volume output for each urination averaged no more than 100 cc, a piddling amount, so to speak.

In the doctor's office, I offered to pee for his observation to display my weak little trickle, but Dr. Williams preferred a more sophisticated test. In his office restroom I urinated into a commode prepared electronically to measure the force of my urinary stream and the volume per unit of time. I was instructed not to consciously strain during the test. After I finished, Matt did an ultrasound examination of my pelvis to gauge the amount of residual urine in my bladder. The study showed that I did have very significant urethral stenosis (constriction) that was "over three standard deviations below the normal," according to Dr. Williams. He reasoned that the stricture of the urethra was probably due to an anastomotic contracture at the bladder neck, a not uncommon, late surgical complication. "But easily corrected," he pronounced with a straight face. Also, I had 50–60 cc of residual urine in my bladder after the test, definitely above the acceptable 15–20 cc for a "normal" man my age, but not enough to be of concern. A larger residual in the range of 100–150 cc could contribute to a urinary tract infection that might further compromise my urethral stenosis.

Dr. Williams suggested that the treatment would be uncomplicated, but would have to be done under anesthesia. It would consist of simply "nicking" the stricture in the twelve o'clock position with a cold knife (as compared to electrocautery) through an operating cystoscope if the stricture was near the sphincter. After that we would try to prevent recurrence by medical tricks and maneuvers to keep the involved area open. Use of the electrocautery unit would be dangerous in the area of the sphincter since that technique could not be safely controlled. Its use might cause accidental injury to the sphincter. Electrocautery would be okay if the stricture turned out to be solely a bladder neck contracture.

Because of the marked degree of stenosis that the tests had shown, he suggested we schedule the necessary surgery right away. Unfortunately, I had planned several important business trips during the next three weeks that would be difficult and expensive to cancel. We agreed to schedule cystoscopy for diagnosis on September 21. The following day, he would correct the stricture under anesthesia as an outpatient. Dr. Williams explained I would go home from the hospital the afternoon of surgery with a Foley catheter in place. He would remove the catheter in his office the following day.

I could tell that Dr. Williams was not pleased with delaying my stricture surgery as long as I requested. I didn't fully understand his concern until he explained what I should do in the event the urine flow stopped completely. "Whatever you do, Jim, don't allow anyone to try to catheterize you or put any instruments into your urethra, no matter what! Probing around near your anastomosis or bladder neck might very well destroy the one sphincter you have left and cause total urine incontinence. Have the E.R. call me, or, if you're out of town, ask them to get a urologist to place a suprapubic tube, and then you get back here to me as soon as possible. Make sure you insist on this no matter how uncomfortable you are at the time."

This scared the hell out of me.

My final trip before my scheduled cystoscopy date was to attend a conference in Baltimore. The earlier trips were one day or twosy's intrastate. I figured I would take them one at a time, and if things got worse I would cancel Baltimore. As it was, I did fine and had no demonstrable diminution in my stream over the next three weeks. Nevertheless, one would be hard put to find a more interested observer of a prosaic body function's performance than was I during this period.

To say I was not looking forward to my cystoscopy would be a very gross understatement. The time between my first cystoscopy as a young medical student and my second a few months before amounted to over thirty-four years. And after my last one I decided that another thirty-four–year interval was minimally appropriate, if not too soon. Nevertheless, I had put the thought of the cystoscopy out of my conscious mind, due in large part to my compulsive attention to my urinary stream. But Monday, September 21, arrived, and I remember wondering what the day would bring. I could have predicted it would be unpleasant, but I wouldn't have allowed myself to imagine the extent of the misery I would experience.

Linden accompanied me to Dr. Williams' office on the chance that he might give me a sedative and I would be unable to drive myself home (or to work) afterward due to the medication. I had intentionally scheduled a meeting-free work day, not knowing how long his examination would take or what shape I would be in after he finished with me. The cystoscopy procedure turned out to be a piece of cake due to what he found, but I was ambivalently relieved and concerned. Dr. Williams had encountered a very tight stricture in the bulbous urethra, the part of the urethra well below the surgical anastomosis and just distal to the external sphincter. He took one quick look and wisely decided not to do any more instrumentation. "That's it," he said, as he withdrew the cystoscope. He did not attempt to advance the instrument through that part of the urethra that passes under the pubis, the anatomical area that makes the procedure so discomforting. "That's all we're gonna do. But

I do want to take an X-ray—a retrograde urethrogram—to see the extent of the stricture and what's above it, if possible."

He continued, "This is in a bad place, Jim. But I need to know if there's also a stricture at the anastomosis and at the bladder neck. An X-ray should tell us that."

The urethrogram turned out to be very fleetingly painful. It required that Dr. Williams manually inject contrast media retrograde into the penile urethra using a 50-cc syringe while Matt was shooting the X-ray. The injection required him to use considerable pressure to force the contrast material past the stricture. It felt like my penis was being blown up like a balloon.

Dr. Williams was surprised at the tightness of the stenosis shown by the urethrogram. The stricture was so narrow that nothing could be visualized on X-ray above the stricture—its length, or whether there was associated narrowing at the bladder neck. I, too, was impressed with the X-ray. The distal urethra had ballooned to at least three times its normal size during the injection, but immediately tapered to no more than a pin-sized opening at the stricture. And very little contrast material passed through it.

I began to worry. I knew that the instrumentation of the cystoscopy and the noxious effects of the contrast material injection would cause the very fragile urethral mucosa to become inflamed. Inflammation is always associated with swelling, and it would take little tissue swelling to convert stenosis into functional atresia (complete closure). "What if... ?" I asked Dr. Williams.

"Well, just come back to the office and we'll put in a suprapubic tube," he answered matter-of-factly.

With that happy thought, I told him we would walk around the area until I felt the urge. When I did, I would assure myself that I could still tinkle before leaving the security of his office. It was a thirty-minute drive to his office from my home in midafternoon traffic.

Linden and I went on to window-shop among the drab medical offices of the area until I began to feel that familiar feeling of bladder fullness. Using Dr. Williams' office john, I was pleased to see that things still functioned, at least marginally. After that, I was satisfied it was safe to carry on with our plans.

The next step was now to go from Dr. Williams' office to the admission desk at Saint David's Medical Center to do my preadmission thing—paperwork and preoperative laboratory testing. My state insurance program had changed since my prostate surgery. Seton Northwest Hospital was no longer a player on the new contract, a typical medical administrative faux pas. Except that I liked Seton, it was of no concern to me that we were using another hospital since Dr. Williams was also on the staff at Saint David's Hospital. He assured me he was comfortable working in either facility.

Linden and I drove to the hospital and I completed the necessary paperwork. I received my instructions on where and when to show up the next morning, Tuesday (5:30 A.M.!), and was sent to the clinical laboratory for routine blood work—and a urine sample. Again, my plumbing performed, although the gross blood in my urine was so obvious that I knew the analysis would be meaningless. Then, Linden and I drove home. Twice again over the next hour after arriving home I successfully tested my urethral patency. The second time, my stream actually seemed a bit stronger. I was elated!

Linden had been tied up with my activities all afternoon and needed to run some household errands. I assured her I was now A-okay, so she left in her car. After thirty minutes of puttering around the house, I felt another strong urge to tinkle. I tried to go, but to my horror, nothing would come out. "Maybe I'm too up-tight," I tried to convince myself, although I knew I was relaxing my sphincter properly. After another thirty minutes of anxiety and increasing bladder pressure discomfort, I resolutely tried again. Nothing! Nought! Zero! Nada!

Linden had not yet returned home. I called Dr. Williams' office and told them I was on the way. I drove my Porsche 911S—my plaything since I purchased it in 1977. The thirty-minute drive took me fifteen minutes. When I walked into the office, Dr. Williams met me and ushered me into a treatment room. It must have been apparent to him by my demeanor that I wasn't feeling too chipper.

"Jim, before we do anything else, I want Matt to do an ultrasound to see how much urine is there to be sure you're not just having bladder spasm," Dr. Williams said calmly. He disappeared out of the room.

Matt went on to set up the ultrasound equipment and did the study leisurely and methodically, seemingly oblivious to my very uncomfortable condition that was now approaching "in extremis." Of course, there was no way he could have possibly worked as speedily as I wished he would.

The ultrasound examination showed a 275-cc bladder size, more than twice the volume I could hold voluntarily since I started measuring my urine output after surgery. I was then escorted from the ultrasound room into a procedure room and asked to lie down on a treatment table. Dr. Williams reappeared and palpated my lower abdomen. "Yep, there's a fair amount there all right," he opined.

No kidding, I thought.

Dr. Williams instructed Matt to set up a surgical tray for the suprapubic catheter placement and again disappeared from the room. Could it be that he hadn't canceled all his other obligations of the day to devote 110 percent of his physical and mental energy to my needs? Doesn't he realize how I'm hurting? Is this all a bad dream?

If I thought Matt proceeded leisurely with the ultrasound, now was like slow motion. My increasing bladder pressure was becoming almost overwhelming. It took all the strength I could muster to lie there without screaming. After Matt had taken an eternity to set up the instrument tray, surgically scrub my abdomen and apply sterile drapes around my lower abdomen, it was another interminable wait for Dr. Williams to return to begin the procedure. Once, I heard his footsteps approaching the door to the room, only to hear his receptionist call to him that Dr. So-and-so was on the phone. His footsteps then sounded his retreat back toward his office. A nonemergency phone call from a patient would never be allowed to interrupt a doctor's patient care, but a physician usually takes another doctor's call immediately. It's a reasonable policy that I followed in my own practice, but at that moment I could have strangled him.

At least five minutes later (it obviously seemed much longer) Dr. Williams entered the room and began preparing himself to do my procedure. When gloved and ready to start, he asked Matt to call his new associate to come into the room to observe the procedure. Matt left the room. A few moments later he reported that the other doctor was just finishing with a patient and would be there shortly. After several more eons passed, he stuck his head in and asked if we were about ready to begin. I was about ready to die! By now, Dr. Williams had shaved my suprapubic hair and further draped off my lower abdomen. After more probing of my tender, very painful bladder, he infiltrated the overlying skin with a local anesthetic agent. He made a small stab incision in the midline skin with a scalpel. Then, he began to prod deeply into the skin incision with an instrument that seemed more blunt than it probably was. My abdominal muscles involuntarily tightened, resisting the probing. After a few more firm jabs, the instrument popped into my bladder with a sudden release of urine into the tube he had attached to the probe. Dr. Williams manipulated the tube in and out several times. This maneuver was most unpleasant. Each time the stiff rubber tube rubbed against tender bladder mucosa, I experienced a most irritating discomfort—like a severe urination urge. But relief from the bladder distention by the urine release allowed me to be so much more comfortable! As I lay there on the treatment table exhausted from my ordeal and so thankful that it was over, I thought to myself that I could surely endure just about anything in the future that might be inflicted on my body. I had successfully weathered this torturous experience without losing my demeanor, and had also kept my dignity intact. I was surprised and quite proud of myself.

After my tube was properly taped in place and a drainage bag secured to its open end, I realized I needed to call Linden at home. When I left the house, I was in too big a hurry to remember to leave a note. I knew she must be quite concerned—I had been in Dr. Williams' office for over an hour (only that long?). On the phone, I explained to her what had happened and assured her I could drive myself home. By this time I was much more comfortable and virtually pain-free, although the indwelling suprapubic Mallinckrodt catheter was irritating to my bladder mucosa. I could feel it rub against the bladder wall with almost any body movement. But, hey, I'm not ready to complain about that, given my vivid recollection of my physical and mental state thirty minutes earlier.

CHAPTER 23

Never a lip is curved with pain
That can't be kissed into smiles again.

—Bret Harte

Linden pampered me at home while I spent an unpleasant evening and seminight. We watched the tube through the evening news, although I have no recollection of what we watched. I was so oblivious to my surroundings, I could have missed the opening salvo of World War III.

I was instructed to be strictly NPO (nothing by mouth) after midnight, but we retired much before that. In my fitful half-sleep I reviewed all the anxieties I had experienced over the last few weeks—some of which I had consciously tried to suppress. The necessity for the suprapubic drainage of my totally obstructed bladder had been a monumental concern, but with its realization, I used minimum conscious thought to replay that experience.

There were two big things now crowding into my mind from some sublevel of consciousness. The first was the possibility that the obstruction represented recurrent tumor. If present, could it be dealt with as simply as Dr. Williams had assured? My other concern represented the possibility he would find such an extensive stricture that its surgical correction would lead to recurrent stricture or complete loss of urinary continence. I was concerned that either of these possible catastrophes might require a urinary diversion procedure. This is an operation in which the ureters are surgically attached to a previously isolated loop of ileum (small intestine) that acts as a new bladder. The end of this loop is then sewn to the anterior abdominal wall skin as a stoma. Like a colostomy, a bag would be placed over this ileostomy site to collect urine, and changed when necessary. An ileal conduit, as the procedure is termed, would demand a significant change in one's life style, to understate the obvious. Only later did I learn that an ileal loop is not a treatment consideration for incontinence in this day and age. Now, there is surgery to replace the urinary sphincter; or injections of bovine collagen (Contigen) have been successful in certain instances.

At 4:30 A.M. I ended all pretense of sleep. I dressed myself appropriately—I thought a workout suit would be ideal—and Linden drove me to Saint David's Hospital near downtown Austin. Again, it was hurry up and wait as more paperwork was necessary—for me and my other fellow surgery admissions. At approximately 6:30 A.M. we were escorted to our room on the surgery floor—a semiprivate room, although my roommate had not yet arrived. I was instructed to change into the standard hospital garb—the famous open-backed gown—and hop into bed. Before I could hop, my assigned anesthesiologist, Dr. Eckert, arrived to discuss my anesthesia. Because he spoke to me in the simplest lay terms, it was obvious he didn't realize I was a physician. No matter, I thought. He was surprised when I asked about having a spinal anesthetic instead of the general he had recommended. He readily concurred that a spinal anesthetic would be safer and preferable. "I usually have to talk patients into having a spinal, rather than the other way around," he explained. "Since your procedure will be so short, I assumed that you would prefer a general."

"It may not be as short a procedure as we anticipate," said I. "But I definitely prefer the safest anesthetic in any case, although it may take longer to wear off." I still remembered my uvular edema from my previous surgery and its horrifying aftereffects.

Shortly after Dr. Eckert left, a hospital orderly wheeled a surgical gurney into my room. He asked me to slide over onto it. After I kissed Linden goodbye, the orderly wheeled me into the operating suite. Then, it was slide over onto the operating table—actually a cystoscopy table—in a very small O.R. obviously used only for urology procedures and, perhaps, minor gynecological surgeries. I couldn't tell for sure, and didn't ask.

I waited. Nothing was happening. Everything had been previously hooked up to me—blood pressure cuff, EKG leads, etc. The surgical nurse wanted to start my intravenous line. There was discussion between her and the other O.R. nurse about whether to wait for Dr. Eckert to do that procedure. The consensus was to press on. I wasn't asked my opinion.

A few moments later, Dr. Eckert came into the room, inspected my equipment and paraphernalia, and spoke to me. "It's Dr. Payne instead of Mister Payne, I understand. No wonder you were so interested in a spinal versus a general anesthetic. Dr. Williams is here, so we'll go on with the anesthesia. I'm giving you some relaxing medicine by vein, and then we'll have you roll over onto your left side and draw your knees up."

At that point I began to feel lightheaded. I have only hazy recollections regarding what happened after that. I remember being turned. I remember Dr. Williams coming in and greeting me in his usual loud, friendly, southern accent. He and the nurses lifted somebody's legs into stirrups at the foot of my table. My head began to clear as I was being wheeled into the recovery room.

I had never before experienced the effects of a spinal anesthetic. It became apparent to me then why it might freak out a few timid souls. The sensation in your body is admittedly weird, but not at all unpleasant. I could touch my thighs and feel my hands touching flesh, but the flesh didn't recognize the hands. And try as I might, I could not invoke movement in any area below my upper abdomen. Otherwise, I felt wonderful—alert, in good humor, absolutely no nausea or other ill effects.

Dr. Williams soon came to see me at my bedside. He explained that at my surgery he had found a very short stricture—less than a half-centimeter in length—in the bulbous urethra. There was no stricture of the anastomosis and only marginal bladder neck narrowing—not enough to try to improve with surgery.

"In my surgery training, one of my professors taught me that 'The enemy of good is better,'" Joe intoned with a twinkle in his eye. He was repeating a choice dictum I frequently quoted to my surgery trainees. "But I easily relieved the urethral stricture. We'll just have to hope we can keep it from recurring," he explained with a big smile.

Dr. Williams answered all my predictable questions: "Yes, the bladder itself was otherwise completely normal."

"No, there was no evidence that any recurrent tumor was present."

"No, I don't know what caused the stricture; although it was most likely an inflammatory reaction from the catheter. Tumor definitely had nothing to do with it."

Dr. Williams continued, "We'll leave the Foley in an extra day and take it out in the office Thursday, instead of tomorrow. During the operation I was so close to the sphincter that I was literally dividing the stricture fiber by fiber. I want to leave the catheter in place an extra day to make sure no blood clots develop to cause us trouble."

After another hour and a half I slowly began to develop sensory sensations progressing down my legs into my toes. After that, I could move my lower extremities starting at my hips, then my thighs, and, finally, my ankles, feet and toes. At first, my ability to move my lower extremities was gross and without control; but I soon progressed to normal, finely controlled movement. Finally, I was wheeled back to my hospital room from the recovery room. I easily slid over onto my bed without aid. The nurses soon discontinued my IV, allowed me to drink coffee, and eventually pronounced me ready to go home. I agreed. With close attention from the nurse and Linden, I changed back into my workout togs and was escorted to the hospital entrance via wheelchair.

Arriving home, I felt a great burden had been lifted. Although I had another catheter in my bladder again (*déjà vu!*), it was amazingly unobtrusive, and not uncomfortable at all for the time being. I guess my penis was becoming accustomed to assault and battery.

The remainder of that day, Tuesday, and all day Wednesday were pleasantly uneventful. My next appointment with Dr. Williams was Thursday, September 24. Knowing I had a freshly operated area of my urethra,

I was apprehensive about how it would feel to remove the catheter. It was very easy. Matt shot an antegrade urethrogram as the catheter was being removed—simply injecting contrast material into the catheter as it was withdrawn and taking an X-ray at the last possible moment.

Dr. Williams was quite pleased at the patency of the urethra shown by the study. If he was happy, I was happy. Then I was fed coffee and asked to loiter until I felt the urge. Thirty minutes later I pissed a stream a horse would have been proud of.

CHAPTER 24

I firmly believe that if the whole materia medica could be sunk to the bottom of the sea, it would be all the better for mankind, and all the worse for the fishes.

—Oliver Wendell Holmes

In the days that followed my urethral stricture surgery, my urine stream remained strong and forceful. Critically important to me, I didn't detect any worsening incontinence. My occasional loss of urine—never more than a few drops—continued to be mild (by my own judgment), and was completely urge related. That is, I never lost urine when I coughed or strained. I would leak a bit only if I didn't find a urinal quickly when the urge to go developed. Unfortunately, the urge continued to develop often, and it rapidly intensified to an almost unbearable state within a matter of minutes. Even under the most urgent of urges, my bladder capacity never exceeded 200 cc, and was usually 100–150 cc, tops. My complaints about this were frustrating to Dr. Williams, also to me, especially when they didn't seem to improve with the passage of time. He explained to me repeatedly that healing of the bladder was slow and unpredictable after surgery. The urgency would eventually improve when the bladder healed from the effects of the surgery and radiation.

Dr. Williams was much more concerned about my small bladder capacity. He worried that the small fluid volume per urination may not be sufficient to physiologically dilate my urethra to allow healing of the stricture area without recurrence.

To help prevent reformation of the stricture, Dr. Williams instructed me to do a maneuver he termed "choke-voiding." Whenever I began urination, I was to squeeze my penis between my fingers just proximal to the glans. This action would partially "choke" the neck of the urethra while straining to void, by that allowing the urethra to dilate. This permitted only a slight expulsion of urine and caused the urethra to dilate proximal to my forced obstruction. It was a moderately painful procedure to do at first, but gradually it became almost pain free over time. Whatever discomfort choke-voiding caused, my psyche completely discounted it. I would have figuratively walked through fire to avoid another urethral stricture and all the associated implications thereof. I continued this trick with each urination for over four months, skipping the maneuver only occasionally—like a sleepy 4:00 a.m. whiz, for example.

Dr. Williams prescribed for me an anticholinergic drug, Ditropan, which he hoped would decrease my urgency and allow my bladder volume to increase. The physiological action of anticholinergics is to relax smooth muscle, such as bladder wall muscle. After two weeks on one tablet twice daily, I saw no evidence at all of the medication's effect on my plumbing. I experienced some expected mild side effects, however. I developed a dry mouth, a little blurring of my vision, and I didn't seem to perspire much when I got hot. Dr. Williams increased the dosage to three pills daily, which didn't change the side effects. After two more weeks I had become quite used to them. In fact, it seemed to improve my far vision. I could follow my golf ball drives further down the fairway (or more often, the rough), and I could read road signs from further away. I really liked the decreased perspiration part. I could run miles and barely break a sweat. If I sat in a warm room or had on too many heavy clothes for the temperature, I could feel the warmth. Even so, I had no concern I would begin to perspire. For the first time in years I could eat the spiciest, peppery foods without embarrassing myself by becoming drenched in scalp and face perspiration. Unfortunately, the side effects were the only actions of the medication I could appreciate. It had virtually no effect on my urinary tract, so I continued to have urgency, frequency, and urine volumes less than 150 cc.

In late November, six weeks after I began the Ditropan, several strange things began to happen. On the Monday before Thanksgiving, I noticed my scalp was extremely itchy following my three-mile jog. In the shower I probably overvigorously scratched the itch during my shampoo and noted later that the vertex of my scalp was slightly sore. No big deal. The next day, however, I had a well-localized, crusted, dime-size scab where I had noted the earlier soreness. It was tender and distinctly unpleasant, so naturally I could not keep my fingers away from it. By the following day I had developed similar crusted scalp lesions on both sides of my head. At first, these were localized also, but by the next morning they had spread to multiple other scalp sites. During these happenings Linden and I had flown to New Orleans to spend Thanksgiving with her sister and brother-in-law. Since I was out of touch with my home medical community, I couldn't readily seek expert medical advice. This didn't particularly bother me at first, but when the purulent crusts seemed to metastasize and multiply overnight, I became concerned. I didn't know what to do other than apply antibiotic ointment to the scalp sores. This didn't seem to affect the process in the least.

While I was experiencing my scalp problems, I developed a recrudescence of what I thought was a fungus infection of the sole of my left foot. Even as my head sores were getting worse, I also began to develop an ulcer of the sole of my foot that apparently was related to the fungus infection. Now my sore foot began to rival my sore head for attention. My foot quickly became uncomfortable enough to demand treatment, so I began warm-water foot baths in Betadine solution, a standard treatment for infection.

When we returned to Austin, I immediately consulted a dermatologist friend who confirmed my fungal foot infection. Secondary to that, he diagnosed a severe infection of the sole with secondary cellulitis and early lymphangitis (spreading skin infection and early blood poisoning). He seemed much more concerned about my scalp lesions. He gave the sores a name even I can't pronounce and predicted a dark future of continued purulence and scabs for an indeterminate time frame. He began me on oral erythromycin therapy for my scalp condition and griseofulvin for my foot fungus. The scalp sores healed almost immediately, confirming to me my own impression that it was simple impetigo, a streptococcal infection common in kids with poor personal hygiene. The fungus infection also responded to the antifungal medication, but that took longer, as I expected.

I'm totally convinced that I developed these problems because of the anticholinergic medication affecting my skin physiology. Its action somehow allowed overgrowth of pathogenic organisms—bacteria and fungi—that flourished due to my altered perspiration. I was never able to convince any of my doctors about my theory, however. Although I enjoyed my hot Mexican food dishes more, and loved seeing my golf ball occasionally land on a distant green, I discontinued the Ditropan. It still wasn't doing diddle squat for my urinary frequency, anyway. I've had no more skin problems, praise God.

CHAPTER 25

The block of granite which is an obstacle in the pathway of the weak, becomes a stepping-stone in the pathway of the strong.

—Thomas Carlyle

Early in November, before I developed the skin miseries, Dr. Williams examined me in his office to evaluate my progress concerning my urethral stricture surgery. Everything was progressing very nicely as far as I was concerned. He agreed. Dr. Williams and I discussed my past treatment, my physical status, and the specifics of my future examinations. As a surgeon with extensive experience in the treatment of cancer, I knew the drill pretty well. Specifically, I knew he would recommend periodic PSA tests, probably every six months or so. I had given considerable forethought to this subject. I wasn't convinced I needed the anxiety caused by having that test on a regular basis for the rest of my natural life, whatever its length. I knew that if my PSA remained undetectable by current laboratory technology standards I was unlikely to have recurrent or metastatic prostate cancer. If the test ever showed any detectable antigen, it almost assuredly would represent the product of active malignant cells, despite how well I might feel physically. My last PSA test approximately three months after my prostate surgery was less than 0.3 nanograms per milliliter. This value is considered "undetectable" by the Hybritech Tandem-E PSA assay, the state of the art standard then. Why not wait until I developed symptomatology that suggested recurrence or metastasis? Why must I sweat out a blood test result no matter how well I feel?

Sure enough, Dr. Williams recommended that I have

biannual PSA determinations. He explained that it would be very important to confirm the diagnosis of metastatic disease quickly. Hormonal treatment would then be started to halt the progress of the disease in its tracks for a variable period. If I waited until metastatic tumor began to cause symptoms—bone pain, for example—the hormone treatment might still prevent the pain from becoming more severe. It would not likely cause any developed symptoms to dissipate, however. For that reason, he explained, it was important for "quality of life" reasons to diagnose recurrence or metastasis before symptoms develop. Because that reasoning made eminent sense to me, I agreed to accept his program.

Dr. Williams suggested we get the first test immediately. I talked him into waiting until after the upcoming Christmas holidays because my family was planning a holiday gathering in California at my daughter's home. I preferred to know nothing either way until after that instead of getting possibly devastating news at Christmas.

While I consciously understood its rationality, the prospect of getting a cancer test done periodically that is so specific for predicting your future mortality was a terrifying one, as I alluded to earlier. Although I had come to grips pretty well with all the possibilities for the future, I hated to think about having my blood drawn. I knew that would spawn a veritable flight of images about the possible results, how I would be informed, how I would react to the news, and on and on and on.

After Linden and I returned to Austin from California in early January, I dutifully called Dr. Williams' office and made an appointment. This was really unnecessary since all I needed to do was pick up a laboratory request form for a simple blood test. That would take less than five minutes total time for either of us. But the importance was in the ritual. Dr. Williams spared me the effect of trivializing the event by having me simply pick up the request slip from his receptionist. Instead, he and I visited haltingly, discussed our respective holiday activities, and then Dr. Williams scribbled the test request form and handed it to me. I took it to the laboratory in his building complex a few doors down the way. A pleasant-appearing, neatly groomed young man in a short, white smock took the laboratory slip and proceeded to skillfully extract a few milliliters of my venous blood without difficulty or discomfort. I had purposely neglected to ask Dr. Williams how long it would take to get the results of the test. As the technician drew my blood, he volunteered that the results of their PSA tests were always available within twenty-four hours. I would know tomorrow what I feared to know, the next day at the latest.

Surprisingly, I worried negligibly that evening and slept well that night. Early the next afternoon my secretary took a telephone call and announced that Dr. Williams was on the phone. Even before I answered I somehow knew he would tell me my PSA was undetectable, as hoped, and that no metastatic prostate cancer cells were active by biochemical determination—at least not this time. I was correct. He told me exactly that. I felt extremely elated for only a few moments. Then, I didn't feel much else, again surprisingly. By the next day I began to think about having to face that same demon every six months. Nevertheless, I thought, today I'm okay. Thank God for small favors!

Although my general mood never scaled the heights I expected upon learning I had no present evidence of cancer cells active in my body, I noticed some subtle changes for the better in my mental attitude. Like any physician, I had developed preconceived ideas about cancer over years of medical practice. Undoubtedly, the emotional trauma of my cancer treatment reinforced those preconceptions. As a result, I may have subconsciously adopted the notion that I wasn't really an active member of the fraternity of life anymore. I probably had mentally assigned myself to some sort of limbo, presuming I would probably die soon. After all, I had cancer! Now, however, with my PSA test showing no present evidence of tumor, my psyche seemed to become convinced that I may have some more life to do after all. As that realization became ensconced, I found myself able to experience real concern about physical and mental problems I had apparently been subconsciously ignoring.

I began to recognize that the total treatment I had undergone definitely had had an effect on my body. For example, I seemed to have had a sudden surge in the aging process. Whereas I had felt previously that I was physiologically younger than my fifty-seven years, I now felt at least my chronologic age both physically and mentally. The morning muscle and joint stiffness I had experienced for years was suddenly more severe and longer lasting. My sustainable energy level had definitely decreased, along with my enthusiasm for new or difficult projects. And I had developed a seemingly ongoing medley of minor ills and other systemic symptoms I had never had before. These things could all be explained by other rationales, but their association with several other physical problems caused by my surgery and/or radiation, or their side effects, made for a much older-feeling Jim. Whether these changes would be lasting or transitory, or would improve with time, remained to be seen.

The verity of the above aside, I gradually underwent a distinct change in my personal focus upon learning that my PSA was still undetectable. Early in treatment I wasn't sure I would even be alive six months after I completed my therapy. With that attitude, my concentration was more to the incertitude of surviving than to what minor or major complications/lifestyle changes I must endure. Now, since I had survived my treatment, and it looked like I may be around for at least another year or so, I became critical again of the banal inconveniences that affect "healthy" people. I reflected to myself that at one point during my urethral stricture treatment the thought occurred that I would gladly accept total urinary incontinence just to survive the acute pain and anguish I was feeling at the time. Total urinary incontinence! Really onerous things seem to be completely acceptable to one under the right bargaining conditions.

First, I resolved to do a better job getting my essential hypertension under control. Linden, like the good nurse she is, had continued to regularly measure my blood pressure, and the numbers were not bad, but not very good. Although she occasionally recorded a pressure reading within acceptable limits of less than 140/90 mm

Hg, more likely it would be more than 150 mm Hg systolic and 90–100 mm Hg diastolic, a moderate elevation. Next, my weight had gradually increased over the last few months despite doing aerobic running regularly. Being a living person again mentally and physically gave me a new incentive to get those excess pounds off. Fat people get heart attacks! My interest in the wellness issues important to a health-conscious person became renewed.

Of course, I did have other problems that were important enough for my mind to elevate to a higher plane now that I was well enough to worry about them. For starters, I hated it that I couldn't even begin to achieve an erection. Although my sex life was not an all-consuming part of my persona before my prostate cancer, the truth that I could not get it up, and may never again, was very weighty on my ego. Although Dr. Williams was absolutely certain that his surgery left the responsible nerves intact, my miserable member had been like a wet spaghetti since my operation. I tried to be optimistic because, according to the medical literature, erection ability may return up to three years postoperatively. The radiation I received was another significant negative for possible function return, however. If another six months passed without some recognizable penile rigidity development, it would be unrealistic for me to sustain any hope for return of spontaneous physiological sexual function.

Somehow associated with the above, I suspected, was a marked testicular tenderness bilaterally. I noticed that the family jewels were unusually sensitive to touch early after my original operation, but instead of improving with time they seemed to become even more sensitive. There was no pain, but I had to be extremely circumspect when washing myself or dressing. They would assuredly reprimand me if palpation was indiscreetly more than gentle and tender.

During the day I now had a "two-hour bladder," just like my friend, Dr. David Wade, who is eighty-seven. Like him, staking out the location of all the rest rooms became my first environmental priority whenever I went someplace. And, of course, I never started a task that couldn't be conveniently interrupted without first taking a prophylactic rest room break. Although I was lucky enough to have avoided the figurative heartbreak of urinary psoriasis called stress incontinence, I still experienced urge incontinence in the worst way. I had to shun light-colored trousers that showed wetness as a dark spot. It was frequently necessary to change undershorts several times on days when I had ignored an early urge or been unable to immediately capitulate to my bladder's demands. At night, I always had to get up two to five or six times per night. In the morning, I would always awake with a moist spot on my sleeping shorts. Several times, notably after drinking alcohol immoderately before bedtime, I awoke during the night with urine-soaked shorts and bed sheets—gross enuresis! How terribly embarrassing! But it taught me to control my nighttime imbibing.

My bowel function was similarly affected. In the past, due to good habits, including a high-fiber intake and active physical exercise, my daily morning bowel movement was always routine, leisurely, and predictable. Sometime after I developed the expected radiation proctitis, I became painfully aware that an approaching bowel urge was not to be ignored or delayed. Simply put, I had lost the anal sphincter strength to overpower my peristaltic urge to defecate. Several times at home I danced a hasty two-step from the living room to an accessible commode while realizing I was losing the battle en route. And only one BM per day was not a predictable event anymore. For a while, a second BM several hours after the first became the rule I expected to live by. Later, totally unpredictable bowel movement was the norm. I might have had zero bowel movements to half a dozen per day, depending on unknown factors.

The threat of diarrhea was especially fearsome. Not only would I urinate in my shorts when I attempted to pass flatus, the flatus itself might be a liquid terrorist in disguise. Having always been persnickety about my personal toilet hygiene, I had used witch hazel pads (Tucks) for years to supplement toilet paper cleansing after BMs. Whereas I could previously predictably clean myself well with two pads, I now had to use six or eight, apparently due to anal sphincter relaxation during cleansing. Finally, eating highly seasoned foods would invariably cause me to develop a perianal inflammation not unlike my radiation proctitis, requiring hydrocortisone ointment for relief. I had never had that problem before, even occasionally.

None of these problems could be considered a danger to my physical health. Taken as a group, however, they sorely challenged my psychological state now that I had survived my first passage through the valley of the shadow of death.

CHAPTER 26

The only limit to our realization of tomorrow will be our doubts of today. Let us move forward with strong and active faith.

—Franklin Delano Roosevelt

Because my PSA today is "undetectable" by current measurement standards, the urological community agrees that no further treatment is recommended for my situation. While this blood test cooperates (remains undetectable), or until metastases (spread) from my prostate cancer otherwise reveal themselves, I am considered "cured" for treatment purposes. This principle is accepted for almost all cancers that are localized at the time of initial treatment. Although there are exceptions, cancers that have metastasized to distant sites are not usually considered curable.

Unfortunately, all cancers have the nasty propensity to recur locally or to metastasize distally for several years after primary treatment. This cancer characteristic distinguishes a malignant tumor from a benign one. For example, a fibroadenoma is a benign breast tumor that can be literally "shelled-out" at surgery and will seldom recur and never metastasize. A breast cancer, however, is treated with much more respect and is, at least, widely excised during surgical treatment. Any breast cancer cells left behind typically may spread to the liver, lungs, or bone. The cancer spread may not be detected until years later.

Fortunately, most prostate cancers grow very slowly. Unfortunately, this slow growth means that recurrences and metastases may become manifest up to at least fifteen years after primary tumor treatment.

Since my pathology report showed that my tumor

had spread beyond the prostate gland into a seminal vesicle, I must anticipate the possible prospect of someday developing metastatic prostate cancer. If I am so unfortunate, the treatment for metastatic prostate cancer today is pretty good.

The driving force for the growth of prostate cancer cells is testosterone, the male sex hormone. Because of this, the best management of metastatic prostate cancer is through sex hormonal manipulation. For decades, orchiectomy (surgical removal of the testicles) has been done for treatment of metastatic prostate cancer because most of a male's testosterone is produced by the testicles. This is very effective treatment, but it has obvious drawbacks. Although orchiectomy is a simple surgical procedure and is still done under certain circumstances, the surgery has now been largely superseded by prescribing medications that effect the necessary hormone manipulation. The medications are at least as effective as orchiectomy and allow the patient to avoid the psychological stigma of castration.

Lupron (leuprolide acetate) or Zoladex (goserelin acetate) are now the treatments of choice for metastatic prostate cancer. One or the other is given as an injection. Either is usually supplemented with another drug, Eulexin (flutamide), a medication that is taken by mouth.

The action of Lupron is to interrupt the normal events in the body that lead to sex hormone production. In the male, it prevents testosterone production by the testes. The medication is quickly inactivated by intestinal enzymes; therefore, it must be given by hypodermic injection to be effective. The depot form of Lupron requires only a single monthly injection to provide uniform action of the drug within the body over that period.

Zoladex is an implant that is also given as a monthly injection, usually into the subcutaneous tissue of the abdomen. It acts by inhibiting gonadotropin production by the pituitary gland. Gonadotropin is necessary to stimulate the production of testosterone by the testes. No gonadotropin, no testicular testosterone.

Eulexin interferes with testosterone at the cellular level. When used with Lupron or Zoladex, it supplements either by blocking the small amount of testosterone produced by the adrenal glands. Large clinical studies have conclusively shown that using Eulexin in combination with Lupron or Zoladex achieved significantly better clinical results than by using either drug alone. In theory, the drug combination should also be even more effective than orchiectomy since orchiectomy does not affect adrenal-produced testosterone.

These drugs are usually very well tolerated and produce few serious side effects. Since testosterone is fundamental in male sexual desire, libido (sex drive) is usually diminished (if it was still present to start with). Some patients may experience weight gain, but that may be due to the effects of the digression of the tumor. "Hot flashes," such as many women experience at the menopause, may occur. All these symptoms rarely require treatment and tend to become less apparent with passage of time.

Treatment of prostate cancer metastases using this hormone manipulation often causes the disease to go into partial, or sometimes total, remission. This is reflected in improvement of symptoms, such as decreased bone pain if the patient has metastatic disease to bone, for example. Remissions may last a variable period of time, often several years.

Although a bad-acting prostate cancer can be rapidly fatal, such is a rarity. Most often it will take several years for recurrences or metastases to develop, and hormonal manipulation can prompt a remission that can last for several more years.

Everything is relative, of course, but in relation to the expected life cycles of most other cancers, the typical behavior of metastatic prostate cancer stacks up very well. Also, it is encouraging to realize that medical knowledge seems to totally replace itself about every five years. This means that new and better drugs and diagnostics are continuously being tested and developed. For example, researchers are now working to isolate a prostate cancer specific antigen. If and when testing for that tumor marker becomes available, earlier diagnosis of prostate cancer may be possible. With earlier diagnosis, better cure rates are sure to follow.

CHAPTER 27

Some things are better than sex, and some are worse, but there's nothing exactly like it.

–W. C. Fields

The physiological issue that was of increasing concern to me as time passed was my sexual impotence. I brooded about my suddenly celibate relationship with my lovely wife, although Linden consistently and vociferously professed indifference to that "temporary" deprivation. She and I had had a moderately active sex life before my surgery—probably "normal" for our ages—but there had been no capability for sexual intercourse since my operation. Nor did I discern any indication that my erectile function might spontaneously return.

In the past, permanent sexual impotence was the expected result in all radical prostate cancer surgery. Recently, however, the anatomical location of the nerves that control erections have been defined more precisely and operative techniques have improved; therefore, many patients now eventually regain the capability to achieve functional erections—usually within eighteen months after operation. In my case, I feared that my adjunctive radiation therapy may have sounded the death knoll to any such fragile nerves surviving Dr. Williams' radical surgery.

Of greater significance, though, was the loss of sexual camaraderie my wife and I had shared before I lost my sexual capabilities. She and I would often engage in harmless sex play when neither of us expected anything to happen beyond the play stage. The important thing was that I had the physical ability to perform the sex act; therefore, the games we played were provocative and fun. Now, we don't do that anymore, or hardly ever, because it's play without a point, actual or make-believe—a sham. This was a difficult pill for me to swallow psychologically.

Linden's attitude, as she expressed in our several discussions, was that she was content just to have my warm and loving (and alive) presence. And although she enjoyed my sexuality when it was available, she could easily wait the length of time expected for my prowess to return. She chose to deny the possibility that it may never return, an attitude typical of Linden's natural optimism.

At Dr. Williams' suggestion, I investigated artificial erection aids, surgical and mechanical; but Linden and I agreed that if sex took that much effort, who could stay in the mood? Dr. Williams grudgingly admitted he would probably feel the same way.

One trick Dr. Williams strongly recommended, however, was the intracorporeal injection of prostaglandin, a potent vasodilator drug, into the penis. Prostaglandin is a hormone approved by the Food and Drug Administration (FDA) for use in babies born with patent ductus arteriosus, a congenital defect. Its action is to keep the patent duct between the child's aorta and pulmonary artery open to shunt blood temporarily into the general circulation. Meanwhile, the child could be prepared for major surgery to correct other life-threatening heart abnormalities. Prostaglandin was also found to cause penile erection if injected directly into the shaft of the flaccid adult penis (probably by the same guy who ate the first raw oyster).

Almost a year had passed since my surgery, and I couldn't even generate a "semi" with the most vigorous urging. "So why not give prostaglandin a try, Dr. Payne?" Dr. Williams urged more than once.

Joe had recently brought two young urologists into his practice group. Both were fresh out of their specialty training and reputedly in the forefront of the latest urological treatments and methodology. According to Dr. Williams, each had extensive experience with the injection of prostaglandin directly into the corpora cavernosa of the penis shaft to effect temporary erections. I knew from my reading that the drug papavarine had been used in the past for this purpose. Its complications—priapism (painful, prolonged erection) and penile thrombosis (blood clots)—limited its usefulness only to the horniest of impotent old studs. When I considered the potential complications of papavarine, I knew it wasn't suitable for me.

Since it now seemed like I might survive this world for a few more years, I decided to try the prostaglandin trick. If it was as simple as Dr. Williams advertised, why not? And I ought to start living again like the alive guy I pictured myself to be before last February, right?

I agreed to meet Dr. Williams' urology associate and prostaglandin expert. He described to me the standard procedure for treating impotence by intracorporeal prostaglandin injection. "We'll start out with a 100-microgram injection of prostaglandin the first time, which is the minimal dose. We don't know how any one individual will tolerate the drug, and if we inject too much, the erection might last for hours, possibly causing a thrombosis of the entire penis," the young doctor intoned blandly.

The small dose suited me fine. Like most other men, my perceived diminutive penis had been a lifelong embarrassment to me, and it had now shrunk further due to disuse atrophy. I assumed his idea of a minimum dose would be approaching my maximum tolerance.

Another concern I had was how to ensure that the medication is injected into the proper tissue plane. The doctor's next pronouncement was not reassuring. "We'll use a 30-gauge needle (which is extremely small) and simply insert it up to the hilt," he explained. "We have to avoid the vessels and nerves that are dorsal (on top) and the urethra, which is ventral (bottom). We simply compress the penis shaft with thumb and index finger to protect these structures and direct the needle at a lateral point."

I tried this scenario in my mind's eye. My thumb and index finger almost touched together when I did the compression bit. My imagined injection impaled my urethra, dorsal nerves and blood vessels, penetrated the full diameter of the penile shaft, and injected the medication into my index finger (which then got stiff).

"We don't have to be particularly concerned where the medication goes within the corpora cavernosa," he continued, "because there are vascular interconnections between all the erectile tissue."

With considerable reservations that went unexpressed, I asked him to set up an appointment to give me my first lesson in penile injection of prostaglandin. At the appointed hour, the doctor seemed unfazed by my lack of sex organ mass as he examined me for the first time. I noted that the 30-gauge needle he would use was indeed tiny, but the attached syringe wasn't. It held a significant volume of the clear, colorless solution.

Explaining again the steps of the procedure as he worked, he gingerly grasped my limp penis in his left hand and stretched it like a rubber band. While pinching the shaft between his thumb and index finger, he plunged the needle deftly into the lateral aspect of the organ. My admiration of his perfect marksmanship was cut short by an intense, burning pain that quickly spread the length and breadth of my member as he injected the medication. Sensing my distress, the doctor muttered dully, "Sometimes we need to buffer the solution if it causes any discomfort. We'll plan to do that next time."

I clinched my teeth and said nothing. He continued the injection until the syringe emptied. Then, he extracted the needle with a flourish, applied pressure to the injection site momentarily, and passed me the baton, figuratively speaking.

"Now massage it," he instructed me curtly, "and we'll see what happens. I'll come back in about fifteen minutes." With that, the doctor moved to the door, flipped off the light switch, and slipped secretively out of the room, closing the door quietly behind him.

I was left lying uncomfortably on a cold examination table with my pants down, embarrassed, hurting, and definitely in no mood to have sex with anyone, especially myself. But I tried as best I could to "massage" what was there. Like trying to pick a worm out of a bait can, my penis seemed to retreat beneath my scrotum every time I let it get away. It became more elusive and more uncomfortable as I continued to gingerly flog it. A few minutes passed that seemed like hours, and the doctor finally returned.

He flipped on the light switch. "Hmm," he said meaningfully, as he gazed at my dead soldier.

"Not much happening, is there?" I proposed.

"Well, there seems to be a slight tumescence of the glans (head)," he fantasized. "Next time we'll use the standard dose, and I'll let you do the injection."

By now it was clear in my mind that injection of pepper sauce through a hypodermic needle (even a 30-gauge) into my former main man was not my personal answer to a sexual dysfunction problem. I knew from my reading, however, that this treatment was generally effective if one could abide the procedure. Also, Dr. Williams had previously offered to give me names of several of his patients who would provide glowing testimonials for prostaglandin injection therapy.

There is no doubt that the prostaglandin injection technique is a valuable tool in selected individuals for treatment of impotence due to a physical reason. It just wasn't my cup of tea, at least for the present. I never scheduled a next appointment.

Today, there are new medication mixtures for injection that cause much less discomfort, are effective, and are quite safe. Maybe I'll give it another try tomorrow. And then again, maybe I won't.

CHAPTER 28

Sex has become one of the most discussed subjects of modern times. The Victorians pretended it did not exist; the moderns pretend that nothing else exists.

—Bishop Fulton J. Sheen

Dear Ann Landers,

I seem to have a thorny problem I don't know exactly how to deal with. My loving wife and I have been married for almost thirty-one years. We have always had a complete and satisfactory sex life and have two grown sons as evidence. For the last few years the frequency of our sexual relations has decreased to a certain extent, but not really abnormally, I would guess, considering our ages.

The problem is, I had radical prostate surgery for cancer eighteen months ago, followed by radiation. Since my operation, predictably, I have been impotent, if I understand the term correctly. What I mean is, I can't achieve an erection. I can still experience an orgasm, although it takes considerable stimulation and effort, but there is no way I can have sexual intercourse with my wife. Although my doctor told me originally that my erection ability might return in several months to several years, it hasn't. I now feel confident that the surgery and radiation effects together have almost surely caused a condition that is a permanent one. My radiation therapist agrees with me. I worry about this considerably.

My wife is very tolerant of my disability—almost too much so. She frequently emphasizes that my impotence makes no difference in her feelings for me and that she can do without sex until my capabilities return. Meanwhile, she won't even allow sex play anymore because she doesn't want to get sexually stimulated. That means to me that we must change our relationship completely and forever since I don't think there will be a return of function. It's very frustrating to me because she wasn't this way before my operation. I think she feels she is being supportive of me by denying an interest in sex, since I can't perform. But instead, I feel even more inadequate because of her attitude.

I have learned there are several potential ways to deal with my physiological problem that should be functionally successful if not anatomically perfect. My wife and I have discussed several alternatives, but she hasn't expressed support for my trying any of them, presumably for the above reasons and, perhaps, the negatives involved with each. For my part, I'm not enthusiastic about injections of papaverine or prostaglandin directly into the shaft tissue of the penis as a way to achieve an erection. I understand that prostaglandin has had good success in causing quality temporary erections that will support intercourse. Unfortunately, I can't contemplate being sexually aroused enough to intentionally stick a hypodermic needle into my penis. Also, a penile implant operation has a few significant complications associated with it that are of concern to me. The operation is also very expensive, I understand. On the other hand, the vacuum suction devices on the market today have improved considerably from early models. I'm told they have been proven safe and effective in producing erections, most often. Although they are moderately expensive, the only drawback I can imagine is learning how to use it and keeping the sexual mood while setting it up for use.

Although my mate and I are not "spring chickens" anymore, neither are we ready to forego the pleasures of sex for the rest of our lives. At least I'm not. The warmth and intimacy that our former sex life brought to both of us were pleasures of living that far exceeded the transiency of the orgasm. I would like to have that again for whatever period of quality living my physical health allows.

Do you have any advice regarding how I can express my feelings to my wife, whom I love very much?

Sincerely yours,
Concerned in Austin

CHAPTER 29

There's a lot of people in this world who spend so much time watching their health that they haven't the time to enjoy it.

–Josh Billings

My physiological functions continued to be essentially unchanged—no better, no worse—for about a month after my misadventure with the prostaglandin penile injection tomfoolery. Then, in the middle of April, slightly over a year after my prostatectomy, my urinary dynamics changed for the better almost overnight without explanation. I ceased having the sudden and demanding urinary urgency and associated inconveniences I had experienced regularly since my surgery. My urge to urinate now developed more gradually by half an hour or more, much as I remembered in years past. My bladder capacity increased to an average of 150 cc, but occasionally it exceeded 200 cc. Although I still had to relieve myself during the night, it was only a single time, the volume was reasonable, and it was never uncomfortably urgent. I still had occasional urine leakage, but that became less troublesome as my bladder irritability lessened. My urinary stream continued strong, and there was no other evidence of a recurrent urethral stricture.

Simultaneously, I noticed marked improvement in my bowel function. Earlier, the demanding, explosive, and unpredictable bowel movements, which I attributed to the sequel of an irradiated rectal wall and anal sphincter, suddenly became much more manageable and considerably less exciting. I still frequently required two sittings, but I no longer worried about loss of sphincter control or other surprises. My anal sphincter remained marginally weak, but not to the extent previously described.

These pleasant and surprising improvements markedly enhanced my outlook on life and my quality of daily living. Although I have no explanation for what caused these remarkable changes to come about, or why they happened so suddenly, I was extremely gratified. I sincerely hope I never have to address these subjects again until I reach such an advanced age that they become the most important part of my daily living!

CHAPTER 30

As long as we are lucky we attribute it to our smartness; our bad luck we give the gods credit for.

—Josh Billings

God knows I don't know what the next year or even the next hour may bring, but I've thought a lot lately about what a damn lucky life I have lived during my fifty-eight years. As a small child I was never cold nor hungry, and I always had a comfortable home and gentle, loving parents. My most unpleasant memory as an adolescent was an episode in which I was humiliated by a peer during a public meeting of adults. This left a small mental scar, but no physical damage.

The worst thing that ever happened to me as a young adult was the suicide of my troubled young wife and the emotional turmoil she and I both experienced before, and I after. That was tough, and it hurt me badly emotionally. Looking back today, it could have been so much, much worse. She might have chosen to hurt our baby daughter, or me, as well as herself. But, thankfully, she didn't.

Except for Becky's death when I was a senior medical student, my life until last year has been characterized by success, excellent health, material abundance, safety, and the ever-present comfort of loving and devoted family and friends. My second marriage, to Linden in 1962, has been as perfect as any marriage could be. It hasn't been free of a few heartaches, but it has never lacked for mutual love and respect. In November, she and I celebrated our thirtieth wedding anniversary. While providing me with unselfish love and devotion, Linden has proven to be a wonderful stepmother and role model to Valerie, my daughter with Becky. Linden has also given me two wonderful sons.

Val caused us both much heartburn as a teenager growing up in the turbulent 1960s—me especially. She gradually straightened herself around nicely and became a successful businesswoman, artist, and mother, to the absolute amazement of this writer. Her four children, our only grandkids, are the delight of their grandmother's eye. Because of Val's skill as a professional photographer, we have followed their physical development well, although we don't get to see them often.

Frank, our impulsive older son, is tall and straight, has no destructive vices, and is becoming a pillar of his Spokane, Washington, business community. Although Frank lacked some needed factor to be successful in academic pursuits (college), he will make it in life because of his good work ethic, his honesty, and his wonderful, outgoing personality.

Jimmy, our conservative younger son, is an Air Force officer and fighter pilot, currently stationed in Korea and actively soaking up Asian culture. His future is extremely promising because of his native intelligence, uncommon good sense and Christian direction. At a time when the family budget was very tight, Jimmy won an acceptance to the U.S. Air Force Academy, saving us the cost of an expensive college education. Like his brother, he is unmarried, but I don't think that will last too much longer for either.

Several months before I developed prostate cancer, the Persian Gulf war began, causing death and destruction to people and the environment in Kuwait. Subsequently, many Iraqi soldiers, NATO allies, and civilians died in that war. Earlier, in my own military career, I managed to miss the horror of Vietnam because I was training to be a surgeon. Earlier still, I was barely too young for the Korean conflict. I was a small child during World War II.

Only God knows why I had been born in the comfort and safety of America in the mid-1930s. I could have been born a Jew in Europe then, as were the six million who died there during the Holocaust. In a twenty-five–year career as a military officer, I never had to experience the horrors of war.

A few months ago the television screens showed the plights of hundreds of thousands of starving infants and children and their families in Somalia. The governments of that miserable country and its surrounding African nations were experiencing the turmoil of anarchy. Human civilization as we know it was nonexistent. It was difficult for me to relate to that situation. I've never personally seen anyone starving. I've never known anyone unable to feed their hungry children. How can parents in those countries abide their children starving to death before their eyes, or dying in their arms?

Today, in eastern Europe, people are hatefully slaughtering other people daily under the sanction of their religion and calling it "ethnic cleansing." Mothers and fathers in the former Yugoslavia must watch their children being blown to bits—killed, maimed, and crippled. Randomly exploding bombs and rockets tear off their limbs and shatter their young bodies. The children must watch their parents being unceremoniously beaten for their religious convictions and randomly killed by impersonal sniper fire. The news media reports stories of gang rape of thousands of young women by the invading armies. Pillage and torture are commonplace occurrences according to the news stories. It was only a few years ago that that beautiful country hosted the Winter Olympics and became a showplace for the world. I've never been called upon to experience that kind of horror or that degree of incivility of mankind to man. Not even close, thank God. I can't even imagine it.

Times are scary in America today, also. Last year, I observed on TV from my comfortable home the riots that occurred in Los Angeles following the Rodney King beating trial verdict. Among other atrocities, I watched in sickening horror as a man was pulled from his truck and beaten almost to death by gleeful rioters. His only crime was to be in the wrong place at the wrong time. I've never even been mugged by a street thug.

We often think we're in control, but we're not. Never was that so evident as it was in the January 1994 Los

Angeles earthquake. We can never escape to a haven of complete safety. The same thing was apparent two years ago in the San Francisco earthquake, and the results were even more devastating. Having experienced many minor earthquakes during three years stationed in Alaska, I know firsthand how terrifying they can be, but I've never experienced a truly damaging natural catastrophe. When Hurricane Elena struck my home in Biloxi, Mississippi, Linden and I were visiting Jimmy at the Air Force Academy in Colorado, so we missed experiencing the full extent of being in a hurricane.

Linden has been a volunteer worker for over three years in the Texas Department of Human Services' Child Abuse Center. The center is a refuge for children who have been legally separated from their abusive parents and are awaiting placement in foster homes. This is a wonderful service, but hearing her tell about the physical and mental trauma children and babies in today's society have endured is sobering and extremely saddening. How thankful I am that my parents were gentle and loving, never abusive, and always willing to sacrifice their well-being for mine!

Typical of her, Linden also donates her time to the Austin Pediatric AIDS League. Here, children with AIDS, mostly offspring of needle-sharing, drug-addicted parents, or sometimes bisexual parents, come for day care while their parents work or receive treatment. These children all die, usually after multiple episodes of painful illnesses. Their deaths are usually prolonged and equally painful. Why? These babies have done nothing to justify their fate. And why must their parents, despite their lifestyle or culpability, suffer the misery of seeing their children die so young, even as they themselves are suffering, wasting, and dying?

As I contemplate all these thoughts and observations, it is impossible for me to feel pity for myself. I have lived already into late middle-age without having experienced any significant physical or mental abnormality or deformity. I've been privileged to watch my healthy children grow and thrive into healthy, happy adults. I've had a faithful and loving wife to provide constant comfort and companionship through thick and thin.

Never have I experienced a painful beating, a serious injury, bankruptcy, loss of a child, jail, serious illness, or being homeless or jobless, save the expected death of my elderly parents, and, of course, Becky's suicide. When my prostate cancer was diagnosed last year, I was truly devastated emotionally, but only for just a little while. With what I've experienced in life and what I've not had to experience, I'll never complain about my fate or future potential for cancer recurrence or metastases. I plan to gratefully live my life to the fullest until I die, whenever that will be. Until then I will be mentally and physically Alive and Well!

CHAPTER 31

The march of invention has clothed mankind with powers of which a century ago the boldest imagination could not have dreamt.

—Henry George

When Dr. Williams and I had discussed treatment of my impotence, he had loaned me a videocassette tape to view that demonstrated the use of a vacuum suction device to achieve an erection. It was a depressing video because the poor guy who was showing the instrument's use was a pitiful advertisement for the machine and the company. He was as homely as a mud fence, skinny as Don Knotts, and was almost as inept at his demonstration as I would expect Barney Fife to be. In addition, the drooping erection he achieved with the device was not what I would expect to be at least marginally functional for the presumed intention. I gave little serious consideration to the idea of using one of those at that time, but, after all, it was quite early in my convalescence. I still had high hopes for an actively functioning organ in a few more months.

Time inexorably passed and I still had no hint of return of erectile function. Then, in May, I attended the Texas Medical Association's Annual Meeting. A most enjoyable and educational part of those conventions is to visit the exhibition hall and contemplate the various technical exhibits. Here, one can learn all about the newest technology and tools of the physician's trade—instruments, sutures, medications—in a "farmers' market" environment.

As I wandered leisurely from exhibit to exhibit, I came upon a booth featuring, of all things, the latest technology in a vacuum erection device for impotence. I showed some interest and the company representative displaying the apparatus was very accommodating in explaining how it worked. The instrument consisted of a hard plastic cylinder roughly two inches in diameter and eight inches long. Attached to the cylinder at one end was a plastic tube that connected to a hand-held pump device that could be activated by squeezing a trigger mechanism. This action created negative pressure within the plastic cylinder. The trick was to arm the cylinder with a constrictive device, such as a rubber band, placed outside the plastic cylinder near its open end. Then, the operator positioned his flaccid penis inside the plastic cylinder. Next, he pressed the open end to his groin at the base of the penis to create an airtight seal. Finally, the vacuum within the cylinder was activated and maintained by periodically squeezing the trigger. As the vacuum developed within the cylinder, blood was drawn into the corpora of the penis shaft and glans, making the organ hard. At the proper time, the operator would deftly slide the constriction device onto the base of the penis from the end of the cylinder, remove the cylinder, and— *voilá!*— functional erection.

The vacuum pump erection gadget being displayed had three different types of constriction devices for consideration. Two were quite ingenious, very imaginative, and apparently simple to use. Standard, heavy rubber bands were the fall-back alternative in case the first two methods didn't work because of some technical or anatomical reason. The company representative giving the demonstration carefully and completely showed me how the vacuum erection device would be used by "my patients." He explained in detail how his machine was so much easier to operate than older models and other suction devices from less innovative companies. I was impressed. He also had a giveaway demonstration videocassette that he coyly slipped into my goodie bag of samples and literature I had accumulated in the exhibit hall.

Later, at home, I inserted the videocassette into my VCR one day while Linden was out of the house. In contrast to the last demonstration I viewed, an Adonis with good body proportions in all important areas was the model. He glided the instrument into functional position with a touch of panache, applied a few quick pumps on the trigger, and, in a flash, he was ready for action. The guy could have starred in a porno flick. Again, I was impressed. I mailed in my order for one that afternoon.

By now, approximately a year and a half had elapsed since my original surgery. Although I hadn't abandoned all hope, I was beginning to see the handwriting on the wall regarding the effects of the surgery and irradiation on my ability to achieve a spontaneous erection. I realized it was still remotely possible that some day spontaneous erections might return, but I was becoming increasingly doubtful. I was unwilling to wait indefinitely for that eventuality if help was so easily and effectively available. Sometimes, use of the vacuum erection device even promoted spontaneous return of function (it said in the brochure).

In about a week my new toy arrived in the mail in a discreetly unmarked package. I couldn't wait to experiment with it, but how? Linden knew nothing about my purchase, nor was I anxious to try to justify it to her. So I stashed the unit in my closet (I hid it!). On my next scheduled trip to someplace, I slipped the unit, which was packed in its inconspicuous, blue canvas carrying case, into my suitcase. Hours later, in the privacy of my hotel suite, I unpacked it and reread the unit's somewhat complicated literature. The instructions were straightforward, but complex, for each of the three alternatives available for the constriction methodology. I decided to try the most-advanced feature first, the so-called SofTouch Constriction Seal. It turned out that the most complicated part of the procedure was setting up the constriction mechanism on the instrument. It required considerable manual dexterity in handling the slippery parts, lubricated liberally with a water-soluble lubricant (supplied). My first attempt resulted in all parts of the instrument scattering noisily to every corner of the hotel bathroom. Fortunately, I had the foresight to lower the commode lid beforehand, or it would have been an even messier fiasco. My next attempt was more successful, and I now had the instrument loaded properly.

Compulsively following directions, I placed my limp member into the cylinder as described in the directions.

Then, I made an airtight seal with the cylinder against my groin. Next, I pumped the trigger to create a vacuum. To my utter amazement, my organ began to rise as reminiscent of my youth. To be truthful, it wasn't this simple. At first, the air seal broke several times requiring readjustment and more lubricant placement around the end of the cylinder. But finally, it was up and, by observation, ready for action.

Continuing to follow instructions, I slid the constriction ring off the edge of the cylinder. It snapped onto the base of my penis with a choke-hold that startled me. It would have caused instant deflation of substance, if allowable, but it wasn't. With that sudden attack of the constriction device, I winced, expecting pain commensurate with the strength of the constriction, but, surprisingly, it was painless. The constriction was functioning.

My erection seemed to remain intact. I had produced what might be a functional hard that was now standing up smartly, as if waiting for instructions to attack.

My next scheduled observation was to see if my erection could maintain itself. I pranced around the room for several minutes, admiring myself directly and by use of the bathroom mirror. Periodically, I tested the quality of the stiffness by touch. After the erection maintained itself without deflating for at least fifteen minutes—long enough for normal sexual intercourse as well as I could recall—I removed the constriction according to the written instructions. What a piece of cake! My experiment was a success, or so I imagined. When I boarded my plane to return home, I was confident that I was ready for the acid test.

Unfortunately, I must have misread my experiment results. The acid test turned out to be a flop, literally. With actual use of the target organ, the highly touted SofTouch Constriction Ring, although mechanically ingenious, didn't keep my erection at a functional level. Although I was barely able to initially effect vaginal penetration with lots of help from my loving spouse, after I fell out the first time, it was like trying to put toothpaste back into the tube. This disaster was softened, so to speak, by the wonderful attitude of my wife. She cheerfully encouraged me to go back to the drawing board.

The second technology was using the constriction rings. These were small, stout, rubber rings in various sizes designed for penis shafts of various caliber. This time, as an accomplished operator of the system device, I had no technical problems with the instrumentation and following the directions. The procedure was similar, but the experimental result of this alternative was even less effectual. It seemed my worst nightmare was confirmed. I had to watch my functional, although artificial, erection slowly deflate before my eyes, even after applying the smallest of the constriction rings.

My last hope for functional success was the use of small, thick, powerful, rubber bands. These were the oldest and "most-proven" methods of constriction. There were two different sizes. Each had an attached "safety release" loop which was actually a piece of string attached to the rubber rings. But these loops were essential, nonetheless, when it came time to remove them.

The instructions advised using two bands at first, and doubling the rubber loops. If two were not effective, one or two more could be added as necessary. Obviously, this method required extensive experimentation and observation. My experiments proved I needed three rubber bands—one large and two small.

After multiple trials and more experiments, I saw why the first two constriction methods had been necessary to develop. Each was infinitely less burdensome than using the multiple, rubber bands—and much less troublesome to remove when the function was complete. It was too bad that neither was a satisfactory alternative for me. Although I found I could maintain a marginally functional erection using three of these very strong and difficult to apply rubber bands, the effort proved what Dr. Williams and I had discussed many months ago: If you have to go to that extent, who can remain in the mood?

To date, I've not had an orgasm using the vacuum suction device, although the mechanics have worked a few times. I'm sure it can be successful for some men. Presently, I just can't personally recommend it based on my experience.

CHAPTER 32

I think that, as life is action and passion, it is required of a man that he should share the passion and action of his time at peril of being judged not to have lived.

—Oliver Wendell Holmes

As I write today it has been two years since this important episode in my life began. The first salvo across the bow in my war with prostate cancer began on a pleasant Friday afternoon in February as I was enjoying a before-dinner cocktail. It is fitting that I will celebrate the end of the writing of this treatise with another TGIF cocktail.

When I began to write this book, I was in the early rounds of my bout with prostate cancer, and I seriously feared for my life. At first, I frankly didn't expect to be on this earth today. That was unrealistic and overly morbid, but the diagnosis of cancer makes one think in those terms. At best, I expected to be in poor health and failing physically due to progression of my disease, or as a complication of my treatment, or both.

There is no doubt I'm not the physically fit, athletically active, sexually potent specimen of manhood I was before this all began. On the other hand, I can still play golf today reasonably well. I'm still able to drive the ball further than all but my strongest and most physically gifted friends. Although I've had to give up my running due to arthritis in my knees, I still can exercise thrice weekly on a stationary bike. This exercise will suffice to keep my cardiovascular fitness intact. I have maintained my work routine without modification, have missed no work due to illness, and travel in my job extensively. Any changes I have had to make in my daily routine or physical activities cannot be blamed directly on my cancer or its treatment. My progressive osteoarthritis has been the cause of what physical-activity limitations I've experienced, and, of course, my almost sixty-years-old body is just that—almost sixty. Otherwise, I feel great!

My cancer has caused some probably permanent physiological changes, none of which are visible, thank God. To me, a very important change is my continued sexual impotence. I'll admit up front I haven't completely resolved that in my mind and psyche. It's a problem virtually to me only, though. Although I didn't believe her at first, my wife is quite comfortable with a noncopulating husband/wife relationship. For my part, I don't miss sex that much unless I think about it, rather when I think about the literal impossibility of it.

As of this writing, I still haven't totally given up on the issue of the vacuum suction device. Maybe someday I'll learn how to use it better. Meanwhile, Linden and I are, realistically, very happy and very much in love. Our marital relationship just doesn't include sexual intercourse. When I fantasize about sex with some cute little sex-kitten, however, I get a sinking feeling inside, knowing I'm truly no threat to her possible seduction—as if I ever had been for the past thirty years.

My plumbing isn't perfect, although it's functional now, and adequate. Periodically, I get concerned about my stream decreasing in caliber, and it may have to a slight extent. Nonetheless, I don't really think my urethral stricture is coming back. And my bladder capacity is virtually normal. I still lose a few drops of urine occasionally when I wait too long to go, or if I pass flatus, but I can live with that. I am very aware of the fact that it could be much worse.

The realistic concern I have about cancer recurrence or metastasis preys on my mind and probably will for many years. As a knowledgeable physician, I know the odds and possibilities only too well, especially that it will be at least five years before I can predict that recurrence is unlikely (but still possible). How much more comfortable it would be for me—right now, in particular— to have the commonly held layman's view that if you survive the treatment, and the treatment was a "success," the cancer was cured. Doctors know too well how unpredictable are malignant neoplasms. Only the patient's demonstrated longevity is an accurate measure of cancer treatment success or failure.

Medical professionals discuss cancer in terms of five-year cure rate or ten-year cure rate. For prostate cancer, a ten-year follow-up is the minimum observation necessary because prostate cancer typically grows very slowly. That's good! But prostate cancer can recur or metastasize ten years or more after treatment. That's bad.

During this phase of my life, a phase I would rather have not experienced, I've taken considerable solace and support from several sources. My medical and surgical care has been outstanding. As a surgeon experienced in academic medicine, I know that the professional competence of my surgeons, anesthesiologists, and radiation oncologists was unexcelled. I'm so thankful that I made the proper value judgments about my healers during a time when panic was probable, and even forgivable. I could have easily opted to seek out popular meccas of surgical care in famous centers and would have received no better treatment than in Austin, Texas. Had that happened, the expense and inconvenience caused to my family and friends would have been extremely wasteful and unnecessary.

Originally, I had concerns about the capability and quality of the Austin hospitals I would need to use for my treatment. I shouldn't have. The physical facilities and professional capabilities were as good as I've seen anywhere.

I had the same initial concerns regarding the Shivers Radiation Treatment Center. Partly by my research for this book, I learned that I had selected one of the best radiation treatment facilities in Texas, both in terms of equipment and professional personnel.

My heartfelt advice to anyone reading these words and facing an uncertain future due to cancer is to seek the judgment of knowledgeable medical professionals, especially your personal physician, if he or she has earned your trust. Ask hard questions about available local talent and resources, and demand frank answers. After you obtain the advice you need from people whose judgment and knowledge you respect, go for it! Have confidence in whatever decision you make.

My loving wife's strength and support during this critical time in my life have been priceless and beyond my ability to express in words. She understands this.

The consideration and understanding of my family, friends, and co-workers have smoothed my road considerably. At the Texas Rehabilitation Commission I'm blessed with a job that is important, personally rewarding, and a very necessary part of the rehabilitation of Texans with disabilities. I know that my being anxious to return to a work in which I take great pride hastened my convalescence. All my associates at TRC are caring, ethical, compassionate professionals who are dedicated to their mission. Their support during my illness made my recovery faster and easier.

I give considerable credit for my present well-being to the knowledge and attitudinal thinking I obtained from several books and authors I embraced during my treatment and after. First, the books by Bernie S. Siegel, M.D., *Peace, Love & Healing* and *Love, Medicine & Miracles*, almost mysteriously presented themselves to me at just the time I was in the most need for Dr. Siegel's message and advice. His experience with the cancer survivors in his Exceptional Cancer Patients (ECaP) organization, and his exploration of body-mind communication and the path to self-healing, were extremely beneficial to me. Dr. Siegel's ideas and teachings were invaluable to help me get my head on straight to fight for my life. There is no doubt in my mind that the limitations of medical treatment are immeasurably expanded in patients who can focus their consciousness on enhancing their natural body defenses. Someday, medical and behavioral scientists will find a way to confirm this premise by scientific research.

On the advice of Dr. Siegel, I became acquainted with *Getting Well Again* by O. Carl Simonton, M.D., Stephanie Matthews-Simonton, and James L. Creighton. I was intrigued by their experience in using awareness and self-help techniques for adjuvant therapy in cancer patients at their Cancer Counseling and Research Center in Dallas. As a younger man I studied Transcendental Meditation and practiced TM for years without apparent benefit. I didn't really accept the mystical premises, although I couldn't deny the documented physiological consequences. After some time I became convinced it was the relaxation response alone that was important. Because of my experience with TM, it was easy for me to practice the relaxation and mental imagery techniques advocated by the Simontons. I think this was especially beneficial to me during my radiation therapy "imaging" my "mad-dog white cells" to chase down cancer cells in my blood stream and elsewhere and tear them to bits. Also, after my urethral stricture surgery, I did my relaxation thing while fingering a piece of soft rubber tubing. I would image my urethra healing like the rubber tubing—smooth and soft and wide. I don't image much today, but I still do my relaxation routine twice daily as mental exercise for emotional/cardiovascular benefits.

Finally, I cried reading Gilda Radner's touching book, *It's Always Something,* which chronicled her sad and mostly unsuccessful battle with ovarian cancer. Ms. Radner contributed considerably to my own mental health by making me realize how much worse cancer affects some, and by my making her strength a challenge to emulate.

Life is so short, and no one knows what delights or horrors tomorrow will bring. These truths are self- evident to most people my age (and totally ignored by most youngsters). When one has experienced the presence of the death angel, even in passing, it reaffirms the fickleness of life.

If my experience can be a positive one and allow me a greater appreciation of the gift of living, it has been worth the pain. Despite my past worry, anxiety, and insecurity of what the future might bring, I have surely come to grips with my mortality and with what I need my life to stand for.

Never again will I curse the weather or throw a golf club in anger. The roses have never smelled sweeter since my illness. My arthritic joints hurt, but I can walk, and play, and embrace my loved ones. I may die tomorrow, or next week, or next century, but I'm sure enjoying today. I'm Alive and Well!

BIBLIOGRAPHY

Altman, R. *The Prostate Answer Book*. New York, Warner Books, 1993.

Anscher, M. S., and Prosnitz, L. R. "Postoperative radiotherapy for patients with carcinoma of the prostate undergoing radical prostatectomy with positive surgical margins, seminal vesicle involvement and/or penetration through the capsule. " *J. Urol*. 138: 1407–1412, 1987.

Boring, C. C.; Squires, T. S.; Tong, T.; and Montgomery, S. "Cancer Statistics, 1994." *CA Cancer J. Clin*. 44: 7–26, 1994.

Brendler, C. B., and Walsh, P. C. "The role of radical prostatectomy in the treatment of prostate cancer." *CA Cancer J. Clin*. 42: 212–222, 1992.

Burnett, A. L.; Chan, D. W.; Brendler, C. B.; and Walsh, P. C. "The value of serum enzymatic acid phosphatase in the staging of localized prostate cancer." *J. Urol*. 148: 1832–1834, 1992.

Catalona, W. J. *Prostate Cancer*. New York, W. B. Saunders, 1984.

Chodak, G. W.; Wald, V.; Parmer, E.; et al. "Comparison of digital examination and transrectal ultrasonography for the diagnosis of prostatic cancer." *J. Urol*. 135: 951–954, 1986.

Committee on Diet, Nutrition, and Cancer, Assembly of Life Sciences, National Research Council. *Diet, Nutrition, and Cancer*. Washington, National Academy Press, 1982.

Epstein, B. E., and Hanks, G. E. "Prostate cancer: Evaluation and radiotherapeutic management." *CA Cancer J. Clin*. 42:223–240, 1992.

Gibbons, R. P.; Cole, B. S.; Richardson, R. G.; et al. "Adjuvant radiotherapy following radical prostatectomy: Results and complications." *J. Urol*. 135: 65–68, 1986.

Greenberger, M. E. *Dr. Greenberger's What Every Man Should Know About His Prostate*. Rev. Ed. Mary-Ellen Siegel: New York, Walker, 1988.

Hamand, J. *Prostate Problems and Their Treatment: Information & Advice for Sufferers*. London, Thorsens SF, 1991.

Hanks, G. E. "Radiotherapy or surgery for prostate cancer: Ten and fifteen-year results of external beam therapy." *Acta Oncol*. 30: 23–237, 1991.

Kane, R. A.; Littrup, P. J.; Babaian, R.; et al. "Prostate-specific antigen levels in 1,695 men without evidence of prostate cancer: Findings of the American Cancer Society National Prostate Cancer Detection Project." *Cancer* 69: 1201–1207, 1992.

Lee, F.; Gray, J. M.; McLeary, R. D.; et al. "Transrectal ultrasound in the diagnosis of prostate cancer: Location, echogenicity, histopathology, and staging." *Prostate* 7: 117–129, 1985.

Lee, F.; Torp-Pedersen, S.; Littrup, P. J.; et al. "Hypoechoic lesions of the prostate: Clinical relevance of tumor size, digital rectal examination, and prostate-specific antigen." *Radiology* 170: 29–32, 1989.

Littrup, P.J.; Lee, F.; and Mettlin, C. "Prostate cancer screening: Current trends and future implications." *CA Cancer J. Clin*. 42:212–222, 1992.

McNeal, J. E. "Origin and development of carcinoma in the prostate." *Cancer* 23: 24–34, 1969.

Mettlin, C.; Jones, G. W.; Murphy, G. P. "Trends in prostate cancer care in the United States, 1974–1990: Observations from the patient care evaluation studies of the American College of Surgeons Commission on Cancer." *CA Cancer J. Clin.* 43:83–91, 1993.

Mettlin, C.J.; Lee, F.; Drago, J.; Murphy, G. P., et al. "The American Cancer Society National Prostate Cancer Detection Project: Findings on the detection of early prostate cancer in 2,425 men." *Cancer 67:* 2949–2958, 1991.

Morganstern, S., and Abrahams, A. *The Prostate Source Book: Everything You Need to Know.* Los Angeles, Lowell House, 1993.

Murphy, G. P. "Report on the American Urological Association/ American Cancer Society Scientific Seminar on the detection and treatment of early stage prostate cancer." *CA Cancer J. Clin.* 44: 91–95, 1994.

Natarajan, N.; Murphy, G. P.; Mettlin, C. "Prostate cancer in blacks: An update from the American College of Surgeons' patterns of care studies." *J. Surg. Oncol.* 40: 232–236, 1989.

Phillips, R. H. *Coping with Prostate Cancer: A Guide to Living with Prostate Cancer for You & Your Family.* Garden City Park, NY, Avery Publishing Group, 1994.

Pilepich, M. V.; Bagshaw, M. A.; Asbell, S. O.; et al. "Radical prostatectomy or radiotherapy in carcinoma of prostate: The dilemma continues." *Urology* 30: 18–21, 1987.

Radner, G. *It's Always Something.* New York, Simon & Schuster, 1989.

Rous, S. N. *The Prostate Book: Sound Advice on Symptoms & Treatment.* New York, Norton, 1988.

Salmans, S. *Prostate: Questions You Have—Answers You Need.* Allentown, PA, People's Medical Society, 1993.

Sampson, A., and Sampson, S. *The Oxford Book of the Ages.* London, The Oxford University Press, 1985.

Siegel, B. S. *Love, Medicine & Miracles.* New York, Harper & Row, 1988.

Siegel, B. S. *Peace, Love & Healing.* New York, Harper & Row, 1989.

Simonton, O. C.; Matthews-Simonton, S.; Creighton, J. L. *Getting Well Again.* New York, Bantam Books, 1980.

Spigelman, S. S.; McNeal, J. E.; Frieha, F. S.; and Stamey, T. A. "Rectal examination in volume determination of carcinoma of the prostate: Clinical and anatomical correlations." *J. Urol.* 136: 1228–1230, 1986.

Stamey, T. A., and Kabalin, J. N. "Prostate specific antigen in the diagnosis and treatment of adenocarcinoma of the prostate. I. Untreated patients." *J. Urol.* 141: 1070–1075, 1989.

Stamey, T. A., and Kabalin, J. N. "Prostate specific antigen in the diagnosis and treatment of adenocarcinoma of the prostate. II. Radical prostatectomy treated patients." *J. Urol.* 141: 1076–1083, 1989.

"The Living Will." *Aide Mag.* 26–27, Aug 1994.

Walsh, P. C. "Radical retropubic prostatectomy, in Walsh, P. C., Retik, A. B., Stamey, T. A., Vaughn, Jr., E. D. (eds): *Campbell's Urology, 6th edition.* Philadelphia, Saunders, W. B. 1992, pp 2865–2886.

Whitmore, Jr., W. F. "Hormone therapy in prostate cancer." *Amer. J. Med.* 21: 697–713, 1956.

Wilder, T. *The Angel That Troubled the Water and Other Plays.* New York: Coward-McCanus Inc., 1928.

Wingo, P. A.; Tong, T.; and Bolden, S. "Cancer Statistics, 1995." *CA Cancer J. Clin.* 45:8-30, 1995

A MESSAGE FROM THE PUBLISHER

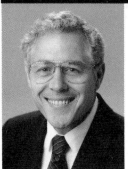

My own family having been touched by prostate cancer, I was moved by Dr. Payne's fascinating and encouraging account of his experience with the dreaded disease. This book is a must-read for any man and any family who must deal with this condition.

W. R. Spence, M.D.
Publisher

RELATED TITLES AVAILABLE FROM WRS PUBLISHING
ORDER DIRECT WITH YOUR CREDIT CARD BY CALLING
800-299-3366

DID I WIN? A revealing, insightful farewell to George Sheehan, America's beloved champion of runners who lost his struggle with prostate cancer, as written by his closest friend and colleague, Joe Henderson.

LIFE ON THE LINE The story of New York Giants lineman Karl Nelson's "fourth and goal" victory over cancer, not once, but twice. Go from the politics and personalities of the Giants locker room to the inner sanctum of the cancer hospital as Karl wins his biggest game—life!

YOUNG AT HEART No other athlete this century has managed to defy the calendar like Johnny Kelley. Eighty-seven years old and still running—61 Boston Marathons, among others. Not just for runners, it is a book for people of all abilities and interests who want to give life their very best.

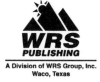

WRS
PUBLISHING
A Division of WRS Group, Inc.
Waco, Texas